T0109521

LYMPH
HEALTH

LYMPH

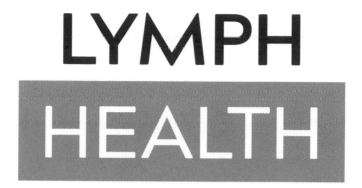

HEALTH

The Key to a Strong Immune System

CHRISTOPHER VASEY, N.D.
Translated by Jon E. Graham

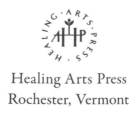

Healing Arts Press
Rochester, Vermont

Healing Arts Press
One Park Street
Rochester, Vermont 05767
www.HealingArtsPress.com

Healing Arts Press is a division of Inner Traditions International

Copyright © 2021 by Éditions Jouvence
English translation © 2023 by Inner Traditions International

Originally published in French in 2021 under the title *Le système lymphatique: Votre nouvel allié santé* by Éditions Jouvence, www.editions-jouvence.com, info@editions-jouvence.com
First U.S. edition published in 2023 by Healing Arts Press

All rights reserved. No part of this book may be reproduced or utilized in any form or by any means, electronic or mechanical, including photocopying, recording, or any information storage and retrieval system, without permission in writing from the publisher.

Note to the reader: This book is intended to be an informational guide. The remedies, approaches, and techniques described herein are meant to supplement, and not to be a substitute for, professional medical care or treatment. They should not be used to treat a serious ailment without prior consultation with a qualified health care professional.

Cataloging-in-Publication Data for this title is available from the Library of Congress

ISBN 978-1-64411-635-7 (print)
ISBN 978-1-64411-636-4 (ebook)

Printed and bound in the United States by Versa Press, Inc.

10 9 8 7 6 5 4 3 2 1

Text design and layout by Virginia Scott Bowman
This book was typeset in Garamond Premier Pro and Gill Sans with Hypatia Sans and Acherus Grotesque used as display typefaces
Illustrations by Rosalie Vasey

To send correspondence to the author of this book, mail a first-class letter to the author c/o Inner Traditions • Bear & Company, One Park Street, Rochester, VT 05767, and we will forward the communication, or contact the author directly at **www.christophervasey.ch.**

Contents

Introduction

The lymphatic system has been misunderstood for some time. Its existence was not really discovered until the seventeenth century.

The reason it has been ignored stems from the fact that, unlike the circulatory system, the lymph system does not have a great deal of visibility. Blood is bright red, making it easy to see and to detect the vessels through which it circulates. In addition, the beating of the heart and throbbing of the arteries can be clearly felt.

There is nothing like this for lymph, however. Because it is a clear, transparent fluid, lymph gives the lymphatic vessels and capillaries a whitish color that makes them difficult to see. Its progress through the vessels is so slow that it causes no surface fluctuations that would suggest its presence. The lymphatic system doesn't have an organ like the heart to pump the lymph, so it has no heartbeats or vessel impulses to invite scrutiny.

Modern studies of the lymphatic system have made it possible to know it better—much better. The further the research goes, the more evident is the fundamental role it plays in body function and its effect on overall health.

Despite its lack of notoriety, the lymphatic system is not only an essential player in the general circulation of fluids throughout the body but also one of the primary components of the immune system. Furthermore, it plays a decisive role in the detoxification of the physical organism.

The multiple functions of lymph make it a key element for understanding the cellular terrain, or environment, and this is why it is of such interest to natural medicine modalities. In fact, one of the fundamental notions on which it is based is that the deep roots of disease reside in the terrain. Dr. Paul Carton (1875–1947), a French pioneer of natural medicine, emphasized this when he said, "The state of the terrain takes precedence over everything." The appearance and development of acute and chronic diseases depend on the state of the terrain, which is the fluid environment of the cells. Depending on its composition, the body stays healthy or falls ill. And this composition is highly dependent on lymph.

The presentation of the lymphatic system offered in this book will show its three major functions: circulation, immunity, and detoxification. It also will show what weakens the lymphatic system and what diseases this can cause.

In the practical part of the book we will look at different therapies that can be used to strengthen and restore proper lymph function. These therapies are quite varied and rely on physical exercise, diet, and medicinal plants, as well as massage and/or toxin drainage.

These therapies are presented in a way that lends itself to application for readers who want to use them either alone or in collaboration with a therapist. In this way the patient can take an active part in treatment and self-healing.

This book, however, is not only for people suffering from lymphatic disorders but also for those who wish to avoid them. It is a very useful guide for prevention.

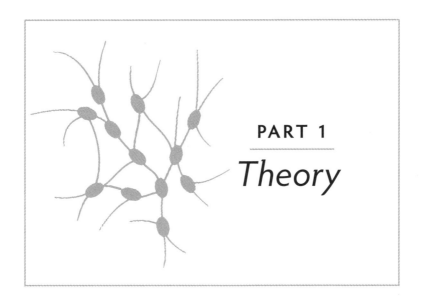

PART 1

Theory

1

Overall Fluid Circulation in the Body

The body is often thought of as a machine consisting of solid gears (the organs) through which a little fluid circulates (blood, lymph). In other words, the body is viewed as being constructed of "dry" and "hard" substances, with fluids playing a very minor role restricted to oiling the mechanism and transporting substances from one part of the body to another.

In reality, fluids in the body are in much larger quantities than are solids.

As we learned in physiology class, our bodies are 70 percent liquid. In a human being weighing 170 pounds, fluids represent almost 123 pounds, or slightly more than two-thirds of its weight. This takes us a long way from the notion of a "solid" body in which a "little" liquid can be found. These fluids are the primary components of our organs: 71 percent of the lungs, 75 percent of the liver, 83 percent of the brain. Fluids are present not only in the vessels but also in and around the cells.

When we talk of fluid circulation, many people think only of blood pumped by the heart and traveling through the blood vessels. But blood is only one of the body's fluids, the one that circulates closest to the body's surface. There are others in the depths, such as lymph, extracellular fluid, and intracellular fluid. Although we may think of blood as the predominant fluid, extracellular fluid is three times larger in volume, and intracellular fluid is ten times larger.

The fluids contained in the body do not mix with each other. They are, to the contrary, distributed in various locations in the interior of the organism.

BODY FLUID COMPARTMENTS

The body's fluids can be considered in the context of their separation in different fluid compartments. Blood is the primary compartment, for it is closest to the surface. It is the first to receive external energies needed by the body, such as oxygen by way of the respiratory system and nutritious substances by way of the digestive tract. Blood composes 5 percent of the weight of the human body. It circulates inside the vascular network consisting of veins, arteries, and capillaries. The arteries are large vessels that transport the blood pumped by the heart throughout the body. Veins are smaller in diameter and carry blood to the heart. Capillaries, which are extremely thin vessels, are located between the arterial and venous networks and form junctions between veins and arteries.

In the compartment directly below the bloodstream we find two fluids: extracellular fluid and lymph.

Blood	5 percent
Extracellular (interstitial) fluid and lymph	15 percent
Intracellular fluid	50 percent

The three fluid compartments

Extracellular fluid, as indicated by its name, is located outside the cells. It fills the tiny spaces, or interstices, that separate cells from each other. The interstices give it its other name: interstitial fluid.

This fluid forms the environment of the cells, the large ocean in which they bathe. The interstitial fluid receives oxygen (in liquid form) and nutritive substances from the blood. It then transports these to the cells, where they will be used. It is also this fluid that receives wastes and residues (toxins) produced by the cells. It transports those to the bloodstream, which will carry them to the emunctory, or excretory, organs (liver, intestines, kidneys, skin, and lungs) to be filtered and eliminated.

Lymph is in the same category as extracellular fluid. It removes some of the toxins this fluid received from the cells and carries them into the bloodstream. The lymphatic vessels through which the lymph circulates intersect with the bloodstream by way of the subclavian veins (starting from below the throat). The toxins removed here will be transported to the five excretory organs, which are responsible for extracting toxic substances from the blood and expelling them from the body.

Extracellular fluid and lymph represent 15 percent of the weight of the body.

The most internal compartment is that of the intracellular fluid, which is fluid located inside the cells. The inner space of each individual cell is quite small, as cells are too tiny to be visible to the naked eye. However, when added together these tiny spaces amount to a significant volume. In fact, the intracellular fluid represents 50 percent of body weight.

The extracellular fluid transports nutrients needed by the cells to the periphery of the cells, where the nutrients cross through the cellular membrane (the cell wall) to enter the cell. There they join the intracellular fluid that carries them to the cells' organelles—specialized cellular parts that have specific functions and are considered analogous to organs—and nucleus, where they will be used. The toxins created by the cells in using these nutrients are then transported in the opposite direction.

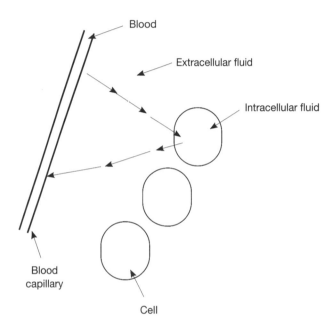

Cellular assimilation and dissociation

The human body, therefore, contains three compartments of congruent fluids:

- Blood
- Extracellular (interstitial) fluid and lymph
- Intracellular fluid

☞ **Good to Know**

The four fluids (intracellular and extracellular fluid, blood, and lymph) form what is known in natural medicine as the terrain—in other words, the environment in which the cells live, similar to the soil (terrain) in which plants grow. The intracellular and extracellular fluids are in direct contact with the cells, whereas blood and lymph have only indirect contact. The quality of the terrain depends on the health of the cells, and therefore so does the health of the entire body.

THE NECESSARY CIRCULATION OF FLUIDS

The body is made up of ten trillion cells. Spread out on a flat surface next to each other they would cover an area of 200 acres, equal to nearly a third of a square mile. Alexis Carrel, who won the Nobel Prize for Medicine in 1932, calculated that to properly irrigate this surface would require approximately 200,000 liters of liquid. However, the human body contains only 50 to 70 liters of fluid, so why don't the cells suffocate in their own waste? How do they continue to benefit from enough oxygen and nutrients?

Such a reduced amount of liquid is enough to maintain life because the bodily fluids are not motionless but rather are in constant movement; in other words, they are permanently circulating. This circulation continually delivers nutritive substances to the cells and removes toxins, carrying them to the excretory organs. The cellular environment—the terrain—thereby remains clean and healthy.

Each of the various bodily fluids circulates at its own speed. Those close to the surface circulate more quickly than those deeper in the interior of the body.

Blood is circulating at a speed of 33 centimeters (about 13 inches) per second when it comes out of the heart and is still fully benefiting from the impetus of the cardiac pump. Nutrient absorption and removal of toxins cannot take place in the arteries and veins because blood flows through them too quickly and their walls are impermeable. The role of these larger vessels is the transport of fluids.

The speed of blood circulation diminishes as it moves into the arteries and farther away from the heart. Once it moves into the capillaries from the arteries, circulation speed is slowed to some 3 to 5 millimeters, or a fraction of an inch per second. The slower speed encourages nutrient absorption and removal of the toxins that occur here.

When blood reenters the veins its speed again increases to about 10 cm per second, which is still only a third of the speed of circulation in the arteries.

Lymph circulation is much, much slower.

? Did You Know?

While the circulatory system has the benefit of the heart to pump blood through the vessels, the lymphatic system has no equivalent organ.

Vasoconstriction of the vessel walls is what causes lymph to circulate. You can get a good idea of how fast—or slowly—lymph circulates by comparing its output to that of blood.

Lymph's output is 2 to 4 liters a day, whereas that of blood is 7,500 liters.

Extracellular, or interstitial, fluid circulates much more slowly than blood because it is not propelled by the heart or by contractions of the vessels. Its speed is still slightly faster than that of lymph.

Intracellular fluid is the slowest moving fluid in the body.

FROM THE SURFACE TO
THE DEPTHS

The bodily fluids don't only circulate horizontally inside each compartment but also vertically from one level to another.

Fluid transfers are constantly occurring among the different compartments. These transfers are essential given the fact that the interstitial fluid is formed from blood, and in turn it is responsible for creating lymph and intracellular fluid.

Let's first take a look at how interstitial fluid is formed. We will have to go deeper into detail here, but this is essential to let us later have a clear view of the fundamental role played by the lymphatic system.

Formation of Interstitial Fluid

The beverages we drink over the course of a day pass through the stomach before they enter the lower intestine. It is in the upper half of this intestine that water is absorbed. It crosses through the intestinal mucous membrane to join the bloodstream and increase its volume. However, the bloodstream cannot retain all this liquid, both because there is limited room in the vessels (their walls are not infinitely expandable) and because this large quantity of liquid will overly dilute the blood.

It is imperative that the excess fluid present in the bloodstream be eliminated. Part of this fluid is taken by the kidneys, which expel it from the body in the form of urine. The other part travels through the blood vessels and capillaries until it reaches the interstitial space.

The walls of the blood capillaries can be easily crossed by chemical substances, such as minerals, or by elements in the blood, such as white blood cells (leukocytes). Their passage takes place through very fine micropores, which are little openings in the capillary walls. Although capillaries are quite small in size, the total exchange surface represented by their walls is enormous; it is estimated at 7,000 square meters, or more than 75,000 square feet.

Filtration through the Membranes

Filtration—the passage of fluids and substances—takes place automatically thanks to the difference of pressure (called hydrostatic pressure) applied by the fluids on either side of the capillary walls. Every time the hydrostatic pressure applied by a fluid on a membrane is higher than that exercised by the fluid on the other side of that membrane, fluid is transferred (along with various substances) toward the side where the pressure is weakest. The fluid there does not have the strength to resist the pressure from the other side of the wall and consequently can be invaded.

This fluid filtration is all the stronger—and the volume of fluid transferred therefore higher—the higher the pressure applied. Conversely, the weaker it is, the smaller the transfer. If there is no pressure whatsoever, no filtration will occur. (Fluid transfers can also be caused by differences in osmotic pressure, but we will not expand on this phenomenon here.)

? Did You Know?

Osmosis is a phenomenon that occurs when two different liquids are separated by a permeable membrane. A transfer of water (osmotic transfer) is made from the least concentrated environment—the one with the fewer suspended materials—to the more concentrated environment. This process lasts until balance has been established between the two liquids.

To have a perfectly clear image of the processes being described here, it is necessary to point out that there are two kinds of capillaries arterial and venous. Strictly speaking, there are not actually two different kinds of capillaries, but capillaries are partially arterial and partially venous. As long as the blood circulating in a capillary is subject to the pressure of the heart's pumping it is called an arterial capillary. As soon as that pressure stops, the capillary is called venous. It now forms part of the venous system that causes the blood to ascend back into the heart without the aortic impulse propelling it forward. Exchanges take place in both the arterial and venous capillaries.

Making the Transfer

Let's now take a closer look at how the fluid leaves the bloodstream to enter the interstitial milieu.

The pressure in the arteries is 35 mmHg (millimeters of mercury), whereas that in the interstitial milieu is 25 mmHg. The difference between these two forces creates a movement of the fluid present in the capillaries toward the interstitial area.

Measurements have shown that in a twenty-four-hour period the blood yields more than twenty liters of fluid to the interstitial compartment. This fluid coming from the bloodstream is called plasma when it is found in the blood vessels and interstitial fluid when it is in the interstitial spaces. Plasma is the fluid part of blood without the so-called figurative elements (red cells, white cells, platelets) and other substances (uric acid, cholesterol).

The twenty or so liters that enter the interstitial spaces blend with the fluid already there. If this addition causes its volume to increase too much for the space, it exerts too strong a pressure on the tissues. This danger is avoided because movement of fluid will take place in the opposite direction, into the venous capillaries.

In fact, the pressure exerted by the vein blood is only 10mmHg (blood pressure is always lower in the venous system than in the artery system). This pressure is lower than that being applied by the interstitial milieu: 25mmHg. Fluid is therefore transferred in the opposite direction from before: interstitial fluid reenters the bloodstream. It can do this easily and with no adverse effects because, being a product of plasma, it has the same composition as the plasma in the blood vessels. This transfer process takes place continually and amounts to more than seventeen liters of plasma a day.

Fluid from the bloodstream continuously enters the interstitial milieu at the same time that fluid leaves this area to reenter the bloodstream.

The seventeen liters that go back out represent a large quantity but not large enough to compensate for the twenty liters of plasma that entered. There are still three remaining liters of fluid that have to be eliminated to avoid congestion of the tissues and organs. A path for elimination in addition to the bloodstream is therefore essential, and this path is the lymphatic system.

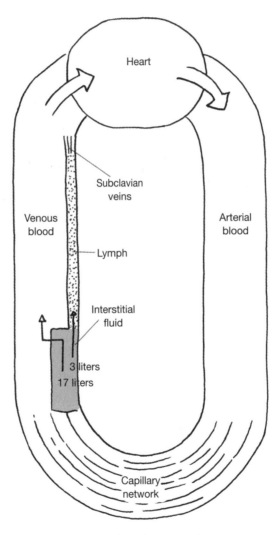

Blood and lymphatic circulation

The many lymphatic vessels distributed throughout the body daily absorb this excess interstitial fluid and transport it to the subclavian veins beneath the throat. There they leave the lymphatic system to enter the bloodstream. This is the way the full twenty liters of plasma that left the bloodstream returns to it. This enables both the blood and interstitial volume to remain stable so that overall circulation in the body takes place harmoniously.

🎓 What We've Learned

- The human body is made up of more fluids than solids.
- These fluids are blood, interstitial fluid, lymph, and intracellular fluid.
- Together they form what natural medicine calls the terrain.
- The fluids are at various depths in the body and circulate at different speeds.
- Arterial blood circulates from the heart into the tissues. Lymph and venous blood circulate from the tissues to the heart (return circulation).

2

The Lymphatic System and Lymph Circulation

The lymphatic system starts in the lymphatic capillaries. Like the blood capillaries, they are extremely tiny (although five times bigger than their bloodstream counterparts). They have the distinctive feature of beginning in a dead end. Indeed, circulation of the lymph does not take place in a closed circuit—that is, with vessels that connect to form a circuit, as is the case with the circulation of blood, which spins in circles. The lymphatic capillaries start throughout the tissues as blind-ended sacs. All the body's tissues (with the exception of the bones, teeth, and nerves) are traversed by a number of lymphatic capillaries that become lymphatic vessels when they converge.

When they join together, several lymphatic vessels form a larger vessel called a lymph collector, which collects lymph carried by many lymphatic vessels. The thoracic duct, also known as the left lymphatic duct, starts a little above the navel and climbs to the base of the throat; it is the largest vessel of the lymphatic system. It measures about 50 cm in length (nearly 20 inches) and has a diameter of 5 mm, which is a scant fraction of an inch. It collects lymph from the entire lymphatic network beneath it in the abdomen and legs, as well as the left side of the upper half of the body, including the left side of the thorax and the left arm.

The rest of the body—the right arm and the right side of the thorax—is drained by the large lymphatic vein, also called the right thoracic duct.

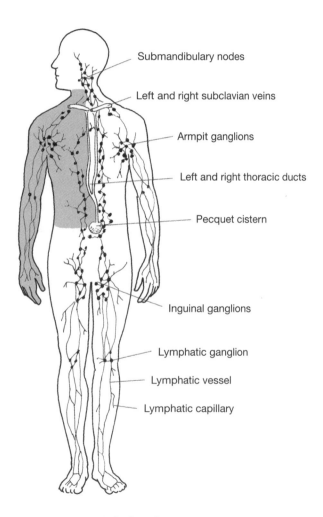

Submandibulary nodes

Left and right subclavian veins

Armpit ganglions

Left and right thoracic ducts

Pecquet cistern

Inguinal ganglions

Lymphatic ganglion

Lymphatic vessel

Lymphatic capillary

The lymphatic system

The left and right collector ducts are connected to the left and right subclavian veins, enabling the lymph to reenter the bloodstream.

The Pecquet cistern, or large cistern, is a reservoir that collects the lymph from the lymphatic capillaries at the base of the abdomen. The Pecquet cistern is located at the base of the thoracic duct and provides it with the bulk of the lymph that it transports to the subclavian veins.

Lymph nodes are clusters of special cells located along the entire lymphatic network and neutralize wastes and bacteria. They have an oval or bean shape and range from one to twenty millimeters (almost an inch) in size.

Lymph nodes are like relays arranged along the course of lymphatic vessels. Several lymphatic vessels can enter a node,

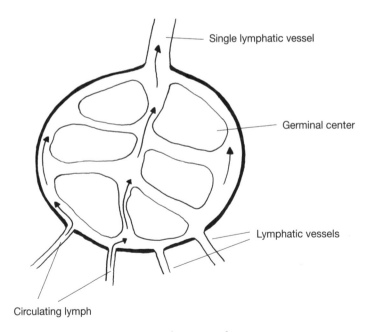

Lymphatic ganglion

but only one will come out of it, and it will be a larger one. Lymph travels through the nodes by weaving in and out of cells called germinal centers, which are microstructures that produce antibody-secreting plasma cells, and memory B cells, also known as lymphocytes, which can protect against reinfection.

☝ Good to Know

There are approximately eight hundred lymph nodes in the body. Some are isolated, but most are arranged in clusters. Many are found in the groin, beneath the armpits, and above the throat (submandibulary nodes).

The lymphatic vessels drain all the tissues of the body and follow paths roughly parallel to those of the veins and arteries. *Draining* is the most appropriate term as the role of lymph is to encourage the removal of a portion of the interstitial fluid and toxins, as opposed to blood, which irrigates and transports elements.

LYMPH

The fluid that circulates in the network of lymphatic capillaries and vessels is lymph. The word *lymph* is thought to be derived either from the name of the Roman goddess of fresh water, Lympha, or from a Greek word meaning "nymph," a beautiful maiden believed to dwell in nature and associated with water. Lymph is made up of the interstitial fluid that has been absorbed by the lymphatic capillaries. Its composition is therefore similar to that of this extracellular fluid, with the difference being that lymph has a higher quantity of white blood cells, primarily the lymphocytes furnished by the lymph nodes.

☞ Good to Know

Because of their similar compositions, interstitial fluid is sometimes also called lymph. In this case it is called *interstitial* lymph, as opposed to the *vascular* lymph that circulates in the lymphatic vessels.

The use of the word *lymph* in both cases explains the different figures that we can find in published literature on the quantity of lymph contained in the human body. Sometimes it is said to be two to three liters, other times ten to fifteen liters. These differences are generally due to the fact that in the first case only vascular lymph is being considered, whereas the second includes both interstitial and vascular lymph.

Lymph is a transparent, almost colorless fluid with a slight amber hue—in other words, very pale yellow. It is sometimes described as "white blood," as opposed to blood that is red. But lymph is truly only white in the capillaries originating in the intestinal villi. The role of these capillaries is to absorb some of the fats found in the digestive process, and it is these concentrated fats that can give lymph a white tint. In the rest of the body it is rather colorless, like water.

THE FORMATION OF LYMPH

Interstitial fluid is called lymph when it enters the lymphatic capillaries. The walls of these vessels are formed of overlapping cells.

Due to the pressure applied by the interstitial fluid, an overlapping portion of a cell can be pushed away from the cell on which it rests to create a space through which the interstitial fluid can enter the lymphatic capillary. The cells of the lymphatic capillaries are like door panels that can open and close. Indeed, as the interstitial fluid enters, the pressure in the capillary increases. When it is too high, the space between the overlapping cells closes. This closing prevents too much of this fluid from entering the capillary and also prevents a reflux of lymph outside the capillary.

The opening of these "doors" is also triggered by signals given by the anchoring filaments in the surrounding tissues that are connected to the doors. They detect any increase in pressure on the interstitial level. The signal is then given to the doors, which, in order to decompress the interstitial area, open and allow the interstitial fluid to enter the lymph capillaries.

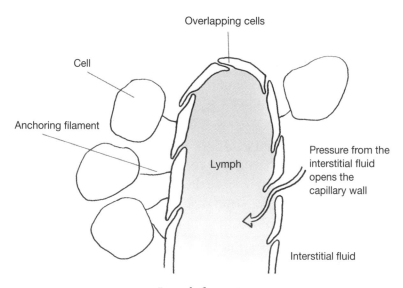

Lymph formation

LYMPH CIRCULATION IN
THE LYMPHATIC VESSELS

While some vertebrate animals like toads and lizards have a lymphatic heart to pump lymph through the lymphatic network, this is not the case for humans. Lymph circulates in the human body by other means.

One of these means is the activity of the muscle fiber distributed in the walls of the lymphatic vessels and capillaries. When muscle fibers contract they shrink the diameter of the vessels, thereby reducing the space available for lymph. The lymph is then propelled forward into a non-compressed zone of the vessel. The alternation of contraction and release creates a peristaltic movement that helps the lymph to move forward.

Another factor that aids lymph circulation is the activity of lymphangions, which act as mini pumps. These are sections in the lymph vessels bordered by two one-directional valves. The lymphangion fills when the entry valve is open and the lymph flow is blocked by the exit valve. The walls of the lymphangions dilate to collect the largest possible amount of lymph. When they have reached their limit, the entry valve closes and the exit valve opens. With the way clear, the lymph, thanks to the accumulated pressure, is propelled onto the next lymphangion, and so on. Because lymphangions are distributed throughout the lymphatic vessels, they enable the continuous flow of lymph. The pumping rhythm performed by the lymphangions can be governed by the body to respond to its needs. The speed of the lymph flow varies depending on the circumstances.

There is an additional way for lymph to circulate: It can be propelled by pressure applied by exterior elements. For

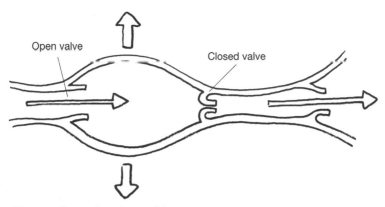

The smooth muscles relax, and the
lymphangion dilates.

A. The lymphangion fills

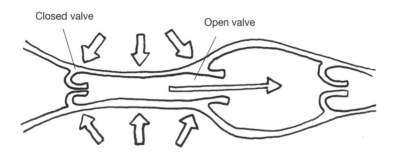

The smooth muscles contract, and
the lymphangion tightens again.

B. The lymphangion empties

example, when muscles contract they increase in volume and
crush the lymphatic vessels with which they are in contact.
This compels the lymph to move. Because of the valves placed
all along the lymphatic vessels, this movement can be made
in only a single direction, that which leads to the subclavian
veins.

✚ Tips and Tricks

All physical activity simulates the circulation of lymph, thanks to the repeated muscular contractions it causes. A sedentary lifestyle has the opposite effect: the circulation of lymph is not sustained, meaning toxins are not cleared efficiently and are more likely to cause problems.

In the same order of ideas, the repetition of the dilation and contraction movements of the lungs also exerts pressure on the lymphatic vessels, thus stimulating lymph movement. Arterial pulses also apply pressure on the lymphatic vessels, as these latter follow paths that are more or less parallel to those of the arteries.

Lymph nodes have no stimulatory effect on lymph circulation. To the contrary, they have a decelerating effect. This deceleration is necessary, however, as it gives the nodes time to purify and disinfect the lymph. The speed of the lymph flow increases again when it exits the nodes thanks to the various processes described above.

The circulation of lymph through the lymphatic system ends after the thoracic duct has led it into the subclavian veins. At this point lymph enters the bloodstream and begins circulating there. The passage of the lymph is made easy as the thoracic duct feeds into the subclavian vein. The two vessels are in close contact, but the fluids they contain do not mix together freely, as a thin membrane separates them. This is, incidentally, the only place in the body where the lymphatic system and the blood system are in such close contact. Everywhere else, the interstitial compartment comes between them. And everywhere else they remain strictly separate, performing their specific tasks parallel to each other.

The entrance of lymph into the bloodstream also takes place thanks to the different pressures the two fluids exert upon each other. Lymph spills into two blood vessels, which are veins: the left and right subclavian veins. The pressure exerted by the blood is therefore weak (contrary to that on the arterial level) and merely 10 mmHg. Lymph applies a higher pressure in normal circumstances and an even stronger pressure in special circumstances, such as a sustained physical effort, fever, inflammation, and so on. The stronger pressure exerted from the lymph allows it to penetrate through the membrane separating it from the bloodstream. Although the volume of lymph that leaves the lymphatic system this way varies, the average amount corresponds to the entry of the interstitial fluid at the other end of the lymphatic system, through the lymphatic capillaries. The lymphatic system thereby contributes in a fundamental way to the steady circulation of bodily fluids. Without it, a link would be missing from the chain of exchanges, and there would be lapses in the transfers of fluids.

Once the lymph—and all that it carries—has made its way into the subclavian vein, it mixes with the blood and is carried farther away into the body. The toxins are filtered from the bloodstream by the excretory organs (liver, kidneys, and so forth), then expelled from the body. The nutrients provided by digestion are carried to the cells to be integrated into their structure or to help their functioning.

LYMPH AND ITS ROLE AS TRANSPORTER

On a daily basis, lymph rids the interstitial compartment of three liters of excess plasma by carrying it into the subclavian veins, where it joins the bloodstream. This is the function lymph performs as a transporter.

Because of the constant exchanges between the blood and interstitial fluid (in the blood capillaries), nutrients enter the interstitial milieu by way of the arterial capillaries and exit by way of the venous capillaries. But just as all the plasma that comes in does not leave again by means of the bloodstream, all the nutrients that come in do not exit again courtesy of the bloodstream. One portion is used onsite by the cells immersed in the interstitial fluid. The unused nutrients are fats and proteins that are too large to reenter the bloodstream through the mucous membranes of the capillaries.

Do nutrients that don't reenter the bloodstream remain useless? No; the lymphatic system puts them into general circulation, as it does with the three liters of plasma. The lymphatic capillary openings are larger than those of the blood capillaries and are therefore capable of absorbing the larger molecules that the blood capillaries cannot.

These larger molecules are the fats released by digestion, such as long-chain fatty acids like triglycerides, which give your body energy. Other molecules are the long chains of amino acids, which form proteins. They can also come from the intestines or be produced by surrounding tissues. These various molecules that end up in the interstitial fluid are absorbed by the lymphatic capillaries, then transported to the end of the thoracic duct. The membrane separating them from the bloodstream there has large openings, so these large molecules can easily cross over into the blood.

To round things off, I should add that large fat molecules enter the lymph system directly from the intestines. This is because in the intestinal villi—where nutrients are absorbed—

there are not only blood capillaries but also lymph capillaries. They are called chyliferous vessels because they absorb chyle, the milky fluid created by the transformation of nutrients in the stomach. It is a nutritious broth high in fats that travels directly into the lymphatic vessels. The more fat the chyle contains, the whiter it is, as is the case with the lymphatic capillaries as well. It is also because of their pronounced white color that the first lymph vessels discovered in the past were the chyliferous vessels. Like all fats, those introduced into the lymph by the chyliferous vessels are carried into the bloodstream by the lymphatic network, which delivers them into the rest of the body.

Lymph also carries other substances such as glucose, vitamins, minerals, enzymes, and hormones, as well as toxins such as cholesterol. Thus, the absorption of nutrients in the intestines is carried out not only by the blood capillaries, as is commonly believed, but also and in a significant manner by the lymph capillaries.

🎓 What We've Learned

- The lymphatic system is made up of lymph capillaries, vessels, and nodes in which lymph circulates.
- The role of lymph is to drain a portion of the interstitial fluid from the depths of the tissues to bring it closer to the surface and into the bloodstream.
- Lymph helps transport nutrients and toxins.

3

Immune Defenses
of the Lymphatic System

While it is common knowledge that defense of the body against attack is the immune system's role, it is not so well known that the lymphatic system is one of the principal components of this system. The lymphatic system includes vessels in which lymph circulates as well as different organs distributed throughout the body. These organs produce the little soldiers of the immune system: the lymphocytes. Large concentrations of these can be found in the lymph.

To further clarify the fundamental role played by the lymphatic system in the body's defenses, I am going to sum up several basic notions concerning the immune system.

Among all its means of defense, this system possesses an army of specialized cells for detecting and destroying invaders—whether these latter come from outside (bacteria, viruses, or plant and chemical poisons) or from within (cancer cells that multiply in a chaotic manner in the tissues).

MACROPHAGES

Macrophages are large (macro) cells that have the distinct feature of being able to swallow microbes and then destroying or digesting them. This makes them microbe eaters (*phage* means "to eat"). Stationed throughout the body, the macrophages intercept everything that poses a threat to the body. When they make contact with a microbe, they adhere to its surface. Their outer envelope dilates on each side of the germ and gradually surrounds it in a circular motion. The microbe then finds itself imprisoned inside the macrophage, in a special pocket called a vacuole, which is similar to a stomach. Once securely stashed there the microbe is attacked by enzymes that break it down into smaller pieces, thus killing it.

Macrophages don't destroy one microbe at a time but rather hundreds of them. They sometimes even combine with other macrophages to increase their efficacy, forming a giant macrophage capable of absorbing and destroying yet more microbes.

THE T AND K LYMPHOCYTES

Among the specialized cells of the immune system are the T (thymus) and K (killer) lymphocytes. There are a very high number of different T lymphocytes, each specializing in the destruction of a specific kind of microbe, and therefore effective against a massive range of possible infections. When infection occurs, the fundamental task is to find the T lymphocyte active against the microbe responsible, then multiply it by millions of copies to confront the invader.

T lymphocytes have receptors on their outer membrane

that easily hold the microbes. They then secrete substances that immobilize them and destroy them with poison.

K lymphocytes also multiply and are programmed to attack specific microbes responsible for infections. They don't poison the microbes, as T lymphocytes do, but instead attach themselves to them and kill them with the help of enzymes. Therefore, they destroy them by *lyse,* or digestion (which disintegrates the outer membrane).

The T and K lymphocytes have to travel to the microbes to destroy them. The resulting combat is not the only possible solution; other lymphocytes are able to poison microbes from a distance: the B lymphocytes.

B LYMPHOCYTES

The long-distance action performed by B lymphocytes (B is for bone marrow) is made possible by the production of substances called antibodies that are transported by blood, lymph, or cellular fluids to the microbes to be eliminated.

Each type of microbe has an outer membrane of unique proteins that distinguishes it from all other microbes. This distinctive marker is called an antigen, because it causes the immune system to produce antibodies against it.

The encounter of the antibody with the antigen kills the microbe either by breaking it down with its enzymes, poisoning it, or causing the precipitation of the organelles of the microbial cells. Another possible action is agglutination, wherein the antibody adheres tightly to the microbe and paralyzes it so that it cannot function.

Antibodies neutralize not only microbes but their toxins as well. This is significant, as in some infectious diseases it is primarily toxins that are responsible for the disorders and physical lesions—for example, in diphtheria, cholera, and tetanus.

Antibodies are produced by B lymphocytes in reaction to an infection, and each antibody is active on only one kind of microbe. It requires a certain amount of time for antibodies to be produced in sufficient number to work against the microbes responsible for the infection, but once they have been created, the body will retain a certain number of them. This means that a large number are always ready to destroy the responsible germ if there is a future recurrence of the infection. A new infection by these microbes is therefore made impossible; the body is immunized against them.

? Did You Know?

The four kinds of cells that are macrophages and the T, K, and B lymphocytes all belong to the family of white blood cells. Their color is indeed whitish as opposed to the reddish color of red blood cells. White blood cells are also called leucocytes (from the Greek *cyte*, meaning "cell," and *leuco*, meaning "white").

White blood cells can be found in modest amounts almost everywhere throughout the body, ready to defend it, because all the tissues of the body can be subject to microbial attack. They only increase in number in a region when an infection occurs. There are, however, other parts of the body where white blood cells are consistently present in large quantities: the lymph, lymph nodes, and the other lymphatic organs such as the thymus, spleen, tonsils, and so forth. The tissues of these organs are high in lymphatic cells (macrophages, various white blood cells). They are produced there and also stored there in large numbers. They also help the white blood cells produced elsewhere in the body—in the bone marrow, for example—to develop to their mature state. Furthermore, the lymphatic organs are where the white blood cells are especially active in their defense of the body.

The close relationship between lymph and white blood cells explains why the latter are also called lymphocytes.

As we have discussed, the lymphatic system includes not only capillaries, vessels, and lymph nodes but also a certain number of lymphatic organs. There is a distinction between primary and secondary lymphatic organs, and given that both are essential players of the immune system, I am going to briefly describe each of these organs.

THE PRIMARY LYMPHATIC ORGANS

The primary lymphatic organs are the organs that produce lymphocytes or, more specifically, stem cells; as they develop, these become active lymphocytes.

Bone Marrow

Bone marrow is the soft and spongy substance that occupies the hollow interior of bones. The stem cells that it contains are the origin of all the varieties of white blood cells. Some lymphocytes are produced in the marrow—the T lymphocytes—but mature elsewhere (in the thymus); others, such as B lymphocytes, are produced and mature in the same place. Once mature, the lymphocytes are transported by lymphatic circulation within the bloodstream to wherever they are needed; in other words, to where an infection has been detected.

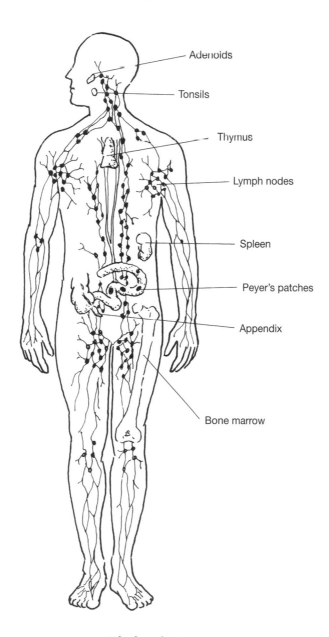

The lymphatic organs

The Thymus

The thymus is a gland located beneath the sternum. Quite large and very active during childhood, it shrinks in adulthood while still continuing to perform its duties. It encourages the development of T lymphocytes. Once they have reached maturity, the T lymphocytes are sent throughout the rest of the body. They are not active in the destruction of microbes when they are in the thymus, only once they are outside of it.

THE SECONDARY LYMPHATIC ORGANS

The secondary lymphatic organs are where many lymphocytes can be found. The environment these organs provide is favorable to lymphocyte survival and activity, so lymphocytes are active inside the organs in question. There they destroy any microbes brought by the lymph or blood, or any other microbes they encounter. These organs are most often located in areas where numerous germs can be found.

It is also in these glands that the B lymphocytes produce the antibodies necessary for the body's defenses, as well as where the selection of the T lymphocytes to counter an invader takes place, thereby allowing them to multiply.

The Spleen

The spleen is the largest lymphatic organ of the body and is located in the left part of the thorax beneath the ribs. We never feel it except when we have run too fast and feel a stitch in the ribs. The pain is caused by spasms of the spleen.

The spleen contains an elevated number of lymphocytes and macrophages that kill all the microbes that are brought there by the bloodstream. It then gets rid of them by expelling them into the lymphatic current. The spleen's capacity to store lymphocytes is very high.

The Lymph Nodes

Although small in size, from 1 to 20 mm (a tiny fraction of an inch to just shy of an inch), the lymph nodes are the lymphatic organs in which the highest concentrations of lymphocytes are found. They are, therefore, particularly important in the body's defense against invasive pathogens.

🖒 Good to Know

The approximately eight hundred lymph nodes in the body are arranged some distance apart from each other all along the lymphatic vessels, but large clusters can also be found in certain regions of the body. These regions are either in the entry paths of the body—the throat, the upper respiratory tract, the intestinal mucous membranes—or at the start of the limbs (nodes of the armpits and groin), where they receive all the lymph coming from the limbs.

The lymph nodes are made of tissues that can produce lymphocytes, but they also contain a large number of lymphocytes from the primary lymphatic organs. They are continuously receiving them as well as adding to them. The lymph nodes, with their active lymphocytes, form the battlefields for killing microorganisms brought by the lymph. Their destruction is facilitated by the fact that lymph circulation slows when it passes through the nodes, thus increasing duration of contact between microbes and lymphocytes and permitting effective destruction of the invaders.

The lymphocytes don't work individually but interact, thus reinforcing the destructive effect of other lymphocytes.

During an infection the nodes that have been specifically mobilized for battle inflate and harden. They can then be felt easily by touch—for example, the submandibular nodes (beneath the jaw) when an individual is suffering from a cold, sore throat, or flu.

Tonsils and Adenoids

The tonsils are small tissues at the back of the mouth and top of the throat that help filter out and kill bacteria that might cause infection in the body.

The adenoids are tissues in the airway between the nose and back of the throat that can abnormally enlarge and obstruct the nasal and ear passages.

These two organs contain many lymphocytes and are like sentries on the entry paths for air and food, intercepting microorganisms that could cause harm to the body.

THE LYMPHATIC TISSUES

In addition to the lymphatic organs, the body also has specific lymphatic tissues. They are small, but their lymphocyte content is high and contributes significantly, especially on a local level, to the defense of the body.

Peyer's Patches

Peyer's patches are small masses of lymphatic tissue, from 0.5 to 1.5 cm in length, found on the mucous membranes of the inner portion of the small intestine, in the ileum region, which is where it connects to the large intestine. The lymphocytes found there detect any invasive microbes brought in by food. They then prepare the necessary immune response, which can be either the multiplication of a type of T lymphocyte or the production of antibodies by B lymphocytes.

The Appendix

The appendix is located in the cecum, at the beginning of the ascending colon, and is a narrow, dead-end appendage that projects 6 to 12 cm from the colon. Surrounded by lymphatic tissue that is rich in lymphocytes, it helps to detect and battle against any infections that enter the body by way of the intestines.

THE ROLE OF LYMPH

What is lymph's actual role in the immune system? Succinctly put, it rids the interstitial fluid of unfriendly microorganisms.

☞ Good to Know

The role of lymph in the body's defenses is not restricted to the lymphatic system but extends well beyond it into the entire body. In fact, the lymph that spills into the subclavian veins brings with it various lymphocytes. They thereby enter the bloodstream, which carries them to other regions of the body where they are needed. In this way lymph takes part in defensive actions in both the lymphatic system and throughout the body.

In fact, the microbes that attack the cells of a particular tissue can be found in the interstitial spaces between functional cells, which are crisscrossed by a dense network of lymphatic capillaries constantly sucking up interstitial fluid. A large number of microbes therefore enter the lymphatic vessels along with it.

Thanks to the high lymphocyte content of lymph, these microbes are attacked immediately. Those that survive the first attack—and there are many when the infection is strong—are guided by the lymph toward the nearest lymph node. The high concentration of lymphocytes there will destroy another number of these invaders. Here again, probably not all of them. But the lymph will carry the survivors into the next lymph node, and then the next, eventually exterminating the bulk of the invaders.

It is possible that nodes will not have the T or B lymphocytes necessary to annihilate the infecting microbe. But collaboration between the nodes works in such a way that those that do have enough will release it into the lymph, which then carries it to other nodes.

So the nodes are not all alike. Not only do they vary in size, but depending on their location and what kind of microbes they face, they will develop different lymphocytes with specific characteristics.

🎓 What We've Learned

- In addition to a network of ducts, the lymphatic system includes ancillary organs: the spleen, thymus, bone marrow, tonsils, and so on.
- The lymph nodes and the ancillary organs produce lymphocytes that defend the body by killing microbes and neutralizing their poisons.
- The lymphatic system forms an important part of the immune system.

4

The Lymphatic System's Role in the Elimination of Toxins

Another major function of the lymphatic system is the elimination of toxins present in the interstitial fluid.

THE TERRAIN

The interstitial fluid is the liquid milieu in which cells live. It forms their environment and fills the spaces that separate them from each other. It is not a simple support but rather a nutritive support that transports oxygen, vitamins, minerals, and all the other nutrients the cells need to function.

The interstitial fluid is not immobile, as it is crisscrossed with nourishing and purifying currents that bring food to cells and eliminate their wastes. It is the vital environment of the cells.

Now, just as a plant can thrive only in an environment that has specific beneficial characteristics (dry or moist soil, limestone or clay, and so on), the same is true for our cells. The cells of our body can survive only in a favorable environment. This environment is called the terrain in natural medicine. It has to contain enough nutrients for the cells and not be overburdened with toxins.

It is normal to find toxins in the interstitial fluid because this is where cells expel their wastes (uric acid, urea, creatinine), but if the quantity of these toxins becomes too large, the body will become sick. In this case, instead of the cells being enveloped in clean and clear fluid, they will be bathing in murky fluid that does not provide a safe living environment.

🖢 Good to Know

Our lifestyle, particularly unhealthy food consumption and overeating, produces a large number of toxins. They collect in the terrain, and particularly in the interstitial fluid.

The overload of toxins doesn't occur suddenly, but very gradually and imperceptibly. Day by day the terrain accumulates toxins, and it is only over time, maybe months or years, that the problems of this accumulation make themselves felt in the form of a disease.

The cleanliness of the interstitial fluid also can be compromised by many unwanted substances other than those the body produces—for example, food additives, pesticides, herbicides, heavy metals, and so forth. Furthermore, every day fifty to seventy billion of our cells die. This amounts to a large number of cell cadavers that need to be eliminated from the interstitial fluid. When there is an infection, the poisons secreted by these microbes and the millions of microbes killed by the lymphocytes will be added to these toxins.

? Did You Know?

Toxins are wastes, such as uric acid and cholesterol, that are produced by the body when it uses food substances. Other toxins, such as depleted minerals and cell cadavers, are formed when the body's tissues wear down. Additional toxins or poisons are substances that should not be in the body and come from outside, including heavy metals from pollution, insecticides, certain food additives, tobacco, and drugs.

Toxins and Disease

The presence of so many undesirable substances in the interstitial fluid cannot help but have detrimental effects on our body, and consequently on our health.

Natural medicine holds that toxins in the terrain are the principal cause of disease (with the exception of illness caused by deficiency). This concept of illness clearly distinguishes itself from allopathic medicine, which believes diseases all have different causes that have to be combated by a wide variety of remedies. Natural medicine opposes this notion of multiple causes for disease and the need for different medications to fight them with the concept of a single cause of morbidity (all illnesses have one root cause: an overload of toxins) and a single basic therapy (all illnesses are treated by detoxification of the terrain).

How do toxins make us sick? They do so in a number of ways. They collect and thicken the blood, which slows circulation. They become deposited on the walls of the vessels (arteriosclerosis), causing them to become inflamed (phlebitis) or clogged (stroke, heart attack). The excess toxins carried by the bloodstream cause congestion of the organs (congested bronchia, pimples, kidney stones), obstructing their functioning (low-functioning liver, renal fatigue) and triggering inflammation (sinusitis, rheumatism, tendinitis).

In the event wastes are not toxic on their own, they still irritate and burden the organs, preventing them from functioning properly. On the other hand, when the wastes are toxic their destructive nature is added to the inconvenience caused by their mere presence. They attack and injure the cells, leaving lesions if not killing them outright.

The presence of undesirable substances in the body therefore has an adverse effect on health. Their elimination from the body is imperative if we wish to retain our good health.

There are two paths of elimination available for these wastes. One is the bloodstream. Toxins enter the blood at the same time as the seventeen liters of interstitial fluid the blood receives every day. Many wastes take this path, but not all, either because there are too many or they are too deep in the tissues. In this case they remain and overload the terrain. Other wastes don't enter the bloodstream because they are too large to travel through the walls of the blood capillaries. These wastes exit via the lymphatic network.

The entrance doors of the lymphatic capillaries are larger than those of the blood capillaries, thereby allowing larger waste molecules to cross through them. These wastes are transported by the three liters of interstitial fluid that enter the lymphatic network every day. If this elimination, complementary to that of the bloodstream, doesn't take place, many wastes are forced to remain in the interstitial compartments with no possibility of elimination. This results in rapid deterioration of the terrain and compromises the survival of the cells.

Whichever route is taken, blood or lymphatic, the objective is to transport the wastes to the excretory organs: liver, intestines, kidneys, skin, and lungs. These organs filter the wastes out of the bloodstream and expel them from the body. The liver eliminates them in bile, intestines via stool, kidneys in urine, skin in sweat, and the lungs in exhaled air.

Wastes absorbed by the blood capillaries that do not make their way directly to the excretory organs do so indirectly, by traveling first through the lymph, then reaching the bloodstream at the subclavian veins.

A large difference exists between these two paths. In the first path, the bloodstream, wastes are eliminated only through excretory organs. In the second path, the lymphatic network, wastes circulating through this network travel through the lymph nodes. These are densely populated by macrophages that destroy all wastes that are interfering with the body, by swallowing and digesting them. This destruction also includes toxins produced by the body, chemical poisons, pollutants, dead cells, and migrating cancer cells. These different wastes are destroyed as the enzymes of the macrophages break them down into tiny particles, reducing their size and neutralizing them. They are thus easier to transport to the excretory organs and, more importantly, filter and expel from the body.

The lymphatic system, therefore, has a powerful neutralizing and detoxifying effect. It provides a significant contribution to purifying the terrain by eliminating toxins. Without it, the cleansing of the interstitial fluid would not be as deep and intense. The body would become quickly saturated with wastes, opening the door to disease.

🎓 What We've Learned

- The lymphatic system rids the interstitial fluid of a portion of its toxic wastes.
- The lymph carries them to the bloodstream and then the blood to the excretory organs.
- The toxins are partially neutralized and disintegrated during their passage through the lymph nodes.

5

Factors That Weaken the Lymphatic System

Proper functioning of the lymphatic system can be compromised in several ways. Here we will examine what malfunctions are possible. In the subsequent chapter we will look at the diseases these malfunctions can cause.

WEAKNESS THROUGH TOXIN OVERLOAD AND NUTRITIVE DEFICIENCIES

The organs of the lymphatic system (vessels, nodes, spleen, and so on) do not benefit from any special status just because they are part of the body's defense system. They are not superior to the other organs but, to the contrary, are dependent on the quality of the terrain in which they are located.

When the terrain is overloaded with toxins, the lymph becomes thicker. Toxins form deposits on the walls of the lymphatic vessels and slow the circulation of lymph. The lymphatic organs become congested with toxins, which reduces their ability to produce lymphocytes. Excess toxins can also trigger the inflammation of the lymph nodes or vessels. This can result in disruptions in the functioning of the lymphatic system and the overgrowth and hardening of certain tissues.

The quality of the terrain is also dependent on its nutrient content. When the lymphatic organs (like all organs) lack vitamins, minerals, amino acids, and so on needed to perform their duties, they become weaker. It becomes difficult for them to produce sufficient quantities of lymphocytes and ensure they are of high quality.

🖐 Good to Know

Deficiencies in the terrain do not spare the lymphatic organs. A reduction of defensive and detoxification capabilities will inevitably result.

EXHAUSTION THROUGH OVERWORK

Every organ is capable of performing its duties properly, if the work demanded of it conforms to its abilities. When demands are made beyond its abilities, it quickly weakens and becomes ill. At this stage it is no longer able to perform its duties.

The lymphatic system can be overworked in two different ways. One way occurs when there are too many toxins to transport and, most importantly, neutralize in the lymph nodes. The other is when the lymph transports too high a number of microbes into the nodes, as is the case with both acute infections and recurring infections.

In both cases the nodes become exhausted and lose their strength and ability to defend the body. The strong activity of the nodes also increases their size. In fact, an organ that encounters strong demands receives more blood, its tissues swell, and its mass increases. While the benefit is that the nodes perform their work with greater intensity, the drawback is that the passageways are crushed. The lymph is unable to pass as efficiently through the nodes, which slows its circulation.

LACK OF TONE
IN THE LYMPHATIC VESSELS

The capillaries and lymphangions (spaces between two valves) of the lymphatic vessels contain muscle fibers in their walls. When these muscles contract they reduce the vessel's diameter, which pushes the lymph forward into the next segment that is dilated. This section fills with the expelled lymph, but when it contracts it then pushes it forward, and so on. Thanks to the presence of valves all along the network, any backward movement by the lymph is made impossible; it can only advance.

The flow of lymph therefore depends on the action of the muscle fibers. As with any muscles, when these muscle fibers lack tone the vessels cannot contract properly and the lymph is not pushed forward. When its circulation slows, lymph can even begin to stagnate in certain parts of the network. The consequence is a loss of defensive and detoxifying capabilities of the lymphatic system.

The lack of muscle fiber tone is caused by poor supply of nutrients due to organic deficiencies in the terrain or a strong concentration of toxins.

Another reason for this loss of tone is a sedentary lifestyle. Normally the contraction of muscles is subject to our will (legs, abdominal muscles, and so forth), and these muscles stimulate the muscles not subject to our will (autonomic) to react in reflex. These muscles are found in the walls of the digestive tract (among other places) as well as in the walls of the lymphatic vessels. The lack of movement in people who live too sedentary a lifestyle deprives these lymphatic vessel muscle fibers of necessary stimulation and thereby contributes to their loss of tone.

LACK OF EXTERNAL STIMULATION TO THE LYMPHATIC VESSELS

The stimulation of the lymphatic vessels and capillaries can come from their muscle fibers or be triggered by external factors.

Every time the tissues increase in volume the adjacent lymphatic vessels and capillaries will be compressed. This forces the lymph to move, and thanks to the presence of the valves it can move only forward. The progression of the lymph takes place more smoothly when the compression occurs repeatedly, because this constantly renews the stimulation. This is often what happens as the organs responsible for the compression—intestines, lungs, blood vessels, and muscles—function rhythmically.

The peristaltic movements of the intestines have an effect on the lymphatic vessels of the belly and stimulate the flow of lymph. The opening and closing of the thoracic cage (essentially ribs) has the same effect on the lymphatic vessels that drain the lungs. At each contraction of the heart, the blood that is propelled forward dilates the vessels of the arterial network. Their increase in size temporarily and rhythmically compresses the many lymphatic vessels there as they often follow paths parallel to the blood vessels. In every action that makes up our everyday life, muscles compress the lymphatic vessels; then when they relax they permit them to dilate. The result of this is also stimulation of lymph flow, which combines with the reflex action of the muscle fibers.

These stimulations are weakened by a sedentary lifestyle, which places little demand on muscles, lungs, or arteries. Conversely, physical activity causes a response in this involuntary peristaltic activity and facilities the elimination of toxins, thus encouraging healing. This is why physical activity is often encouraged by health care providers.

ACUTE INFLAMMATION

Inflammation is a localized defensive reaction that is generally revealed by swelling of the attacked tissues. This swelling (from the influx of interstitial fluid) and reddening (from the inflow of blood) are the two major characteristics of inflammation. The purpose of this arrival of additional liquid in the stricken region is to facilitate the transport of lymphocytes necessary to fight the aggressive activity of microbes or toxic substances.

There is a drawback to this swelling of the tissues, however. The lymphatic vessels in this area no longer have as much space at their disposal and are compressed, which sharply curtails the circulation of the lymph. This continuous compression will last for as long as the area remains inflamed.

So, while blood circulation is accelerated, lymph circulation slows to a crawl and can even come to a complete halt upstream of the clog. The resulting stasis leads to an accumulation of toxins and dead microbes that, because they are not being drained, irritate and attack the lymphatic vessels.

☞ Good to Know

While acute inflammations need to be left alone to do their beneficial work, we must guard against chronic inflammation, which will hinder lymph circulation over the long term.

ACUTE INFECTION

In an acute infection, an enormous number of germs need to be neutralized. The lymph nodes in the stricken region consequently labor intensively to destroy them and to produce new lymphocytes.

This dual activity of the lymph nodes causes an increase in their size for two reasons: more blood is irrigating them, and the number of lymphocytes stored in their tissues is increasing. The increased size forces the nodes to dilate and compresses the paths of lymph circulation, which now slows and even stagnates. The region of the body will then no longer benefit from as large an influx of lymphocytes, nor will it benefit from the detoxifying activity of the lymphatic system. This problem is only temporary; once the infection has been overcome, the nodes go back to their normal size and the normal flow of lymph is restored.

MECHANICAL OBSTACLES

Along the same idea, a tumor, lump, or cyst in close proximity or direct contact with a lymph node or vessel will apply pressure to it. The progression of lymph will be hindered in proportion to the pressure exerted. This is especially true when a tumor develops in the walls of the lymphatic vessels or nodes.

INJURIES TO
THE LYMPHATIC VESSELS

The lymphatic vessels and capillaries are extremely thin and delicate. Therefore, those located near the surface of the skin can easily be injured. Such injuries occur when someone has a wound or scrape, crushes and tears tissues, gets hit accidentally with a hammer, walks into a piece of furniture, and so forth. These injuries inevitably occur during surgical operations and radiation treatments.

In such cases, the walls of certain lymphatic vessels are partially destroyed and no longer able to retain the lymph, which then flows outside of the vessels. This is not an incurable problem. The lymphatic vessels have the ability to regenerate and restore contact with the injured part of the vessel or to lengthen the still-functioning portion of the vessel, which will advance its way into the non-irrigated tissues.

REMOVAL OF THE NODES

In addition to being a path for the elimination of toxins, the lymphatic network also transports cells. Among these we find beneficial lymphocytes as well as cells that are harmful to the body, such as cancer cells.

Cancer cells can be carried by the lymph from their place of origin (the tumor) to another region of the body. There, when circumstances permit, they will attach themselves and multiply, forming a new tumor (metastasis). To prevent this from happening, when a tumor is surgically removed the adjacent lymph nodes will be removed. For example, during breast cancer surgery the axillary (armpit) nodes can also be removed so that lymph that transits through these nodes to enter the arms can no longer do so. The disadvantage of this intervention is, however, that lymph in the arm will now have a more difficult time leaving and may collect and cause lymphedema (fluid buildup).

? Did You Know?

The removal of tonsils or appendix won't cause lymphedema because these tissues are high in lymphatic cells and not crossed by the flow of lymph, as is the case for the nodes.

DEHYDRATION

When the daily quantity of liquid supplied to the body is insufficient, blood flow diminishes and slows lymphatic circulation. This is because the reduction of blood volume reduces the blood's pressure on the blood capillaries, which reduces the formation of interstitial fluid and its passage into the lymphatic system. In fact, the circulation of lymph is partially dependent on the impetus given it by the interstitial fluid entering it. When this impetus is weakened, the lymph circulates more slowly than it should.

The bottom line is that the speed with which lymph circulates depends greatly on blood pressure. However, while it is quite difficult to act directly on lymphatic circulation, it is very simple to do so indirectly. All it takes is to increase the blood pressure—for example, by a hydration cure. The same effect can be achieved through physical exercise.

POOR VEIN CIRCULATION

Some people have poor blood circulation in their veins, so the blood has a tendency to stagnate and thicken. The pressure exerted by the venous blood on the vein capillaries is then higher than it would be normally. Because the daily passage of seventeen liters of interstitial fluid through the walls of the venous capillaries depends on higher pressure from the interstitial side, the increased pressure on the venous side reduces the difference between the two pressures and thereby reduces the passage of interstitial fluid into the venous system.

The consequence of this is that many toxins that would have been carried away by the venous blood are not. Instead they remain in the interstitial fluid, where they collect. Because these surplus toxins are not being evacuated by way of the venous system, the lymphatic system will have to take responsibility for removing them. Over time, this extra work depletes and weakens it.

🎓 What We've Learned

The principal causes of a weakened lymphatic system are:

- A terrain overloaded with toxins
- Sedentary lifestyle
- Poor venous circulation
- Lack of muscle tone in the walls of the lymphatic vessels
- Removal of nodes
- Deficiencies in liquids and nutrients

6

Diseases of the Lymphatic System

The weakening of the lymphatic system disrupts its functioning and can result in numerous diseases. These are all connected to the three main functions of the lymphatic system: its circulation, immune system, and detoxifying functions.

CIRCULATORY DISEASES

There are several types of diseases that can be classified as circulatory.

Lymphedema

Lymphedema is a long-term swelling of a part of the body and is caused by an accumulation of lymph. The most common locations are the arms and legs, and more rarely the face, throat, and abdomen. The swelling of the limbs can be partial or total. For example, it may be only an ankle or it may be both ankles and the entire leg; it can affect a single limb or both.

Swelling of the tissues is caused when an obstacle blocks the circulation of the lymph. It is no longer able to move forward and stagnates in the lymphatic vessels. The interstitial fluid is then prevented from entering the lymphatic network and accumulates in the interstitial space around the cells of the afflicted part of the body. Over time this accumulation of fluid increases the volume of the tissues.

The term *lymphedema* is justified even though the swelling is caused primarily by the interstitial fluid. In fact, this fluid is also known as interstitial lymph. The edema is therefore clearly caused by lymph. Furthermore, when the pressure inside the lymphatic vessels becomes too high—because of the blocked circulation of lymph—part of the lymph they contain is pushed outside of the lymphatic capillaries, something that never happens normally. This lymph then combines with the interstitial lymph.

We can compare the formation of an edema to a traffic jam. While the circulation of cars on the road network is normally fluid, all it takes is an accident blocking the main highway for all the areas it serves to become congested with vehicles.

The causes for the blockage of lymph circulation are multiple. Most often, a portion of the structure of the lymph nodes, capillaries, or vessels has been heavily damaged, either by an injury, surgical operation, or radiation treatment. The resulting destruction of the vessels prevents the lymph from moving forward normally.

Another cause can be the rips, lesions, and infections that can sometimes germinate at the formation of overly thick scar tissue. These latter block the free passage of the lymphatic vessels and capillaries, thereby obstructing the circulation of lymph. The obstruction of the lymphatic plumbing can also be due to the presence of a tumor that compresses the lymphatic vessels and thereby opposes the lymph's continued progress.

Any removal of the nodes also prevents lymph circulation from occurring properly. When the path it needed to take to continue on its way has been destroyed, lymph can no longer move forward. It then will spill into the tissues and collect.

There are two functional causes that can be added to these injury-related causes. The first is poor venous circulation, which slows the passage of the seventeen liters of interstitial fluid that has to go back into the bloodstream every day, meaning some remains in the interstitial space and leads to swelling of the tissues. The second function-related cause is the lack of physical exercise. Sedentary behavior reduces muscle tone in general, thus also that of the muscles in the lymphatic vessels, which play such an important role in the progression of lymph.

🖐 Good to Know

Weaknesses of the lymphatic system responsible for lymphedema can be congenital, but most often this swelling is caused by poor lifestyle or as a side effect of surgery.

Studies have shown that 20 to 30 percent of women suffering from lymphedema were stricken following a breast cancer operation (with removal of the axillary lymph nodes to prevent metastasis) and radiation therapy treatment.

When the cause is lifestyle, formation of lymphedema is gradual:

- In the first stage the edema is present only during the day. When the swollen region is lightly pressed, a slight depression persists for a little while after the pressure is removed. At this stage, raising the limb causes the edema to disappear more or less completely. Rest from a good night's sleep has the same effect.

- In the second stage neither rest nor raising the limb will cause the swelling to disappear. It is therefore present day and night. The tissues have hardened, and it is quite difficult or impossible to press an impression into the skin. Furthermore, the accumulation of fluid at skin level erases the wrinkles and bumps that normally can be seen over the joints, muscles, and blood vessels. For example, the back of the hands no longer have any definition but have become smooth surfaces.

- In the third stage, if the illness continues to progress, there is a thickening of the skin and greater vulnerability to infection. The circulation of lymph at the cutaneous level has become so weak that there are few lymphocytes to offer protection against infection. Aggravating the situation, the undrained toxins accumulating in the area offer germs an ideal terrain for multiplying.

? Did You Know?

Swollen ankles are not always caused by a lymphatic system disorder. Overconsumption of salt may be responsible, because salt retains fluid in the tissues (1 gram of salt will retain 11 grams of water). Cardiac weakness is another cause. A tired heart cannot pump fluids with enough strength, so they stagnate in the lower levels of the body, and interstitial fluid accumulates at the ankles.

The swelling of a limb, for example a leg, creates a more or less constant irritation with a sensation of heaviness or perhaps pain. It also restricts mobility; the limbs are more difficult to use, and certain movements are no longer possible. Lymphedema is a handicapping disease.

Weight Gain

Gaining weight has a variety of possible causes, but one is deficient lymphatic circulation. This is because among its many roles, lymph also transports fats.

The fats provided by the digestive process have two ways to make their way to the tissues where they will be used. One portion enters the bloodstream and is carried to the liver to be transformed before traveling farther on its journey. These fat molecules are small in size, as is generally the case with all molecules transported by the bloodstream. The other portion of fats doesn't enter the blood but instead goes directly into the lymphatic network at the level of the intestinal capillaries (the lacteals). The lymph then carries it up to the subclavian veins, where it enters the bloodstream. These are primarily large fat molecules, consequently the ones that are more difficult to use and digest.

So we see that the large fat molecules have to be transported by lymphatic circulation, but when lymph circulation is poor and the vessels congested, their walls can rupture. Lymph, and the large fat molecules it contains, then spill into the interstitial fluid, putting these molecules in close contact with the cells of the surrounding tissues. Among these cells are adipocytes, cells specializing in the storage of fats and that are found in practically all body tissues. They are like pouches that not only become filled with fat but can also dilate to increase their storage capacity. Their walls are therefore expandable.

Adipocytes are small in size, but there are many of them. When a number of them dilate they increase the size of the adipose (fatty) tissues. Cellulite formation and weight gain are the inevitable results. These problems would not have occurred if lymphatic circulation had not been hampered. In fact, the fats that the lymph was transporting would not have left the lymphatic network to enter into the interstitial compartment and become stored in the adipocytes.

General Circulation Problems

The lymphatic system alone does not bear all the consequences of poor circulation caused by stasis and obstructions. It is not isolated; it's closely connected to the overall circulation system, which also includes the bloodstream. The consequence of the close interdependence of blood circulation and lymphatic circulation means that any disruption of one will have repercussions on the other.

When lymph circulates more slowly, the three liters of interstitial fluid it is intended to absorb and carry into the bloodstream (via the subclavian veins) does not reach the blood, or at least not in sufficient quantity. This supply of liquid is therefore missing from the bloodstream. The change in blood volume then disrupts the balance between arterial blood and venous blood.

What is going to happen to these three liters of interstitial fluid that have been incompletely or not at all absorbed by the lymphatic capillaries?

Because the lymphatic circulation is deficient, venous blood has to do its job instead. Now, if one or two liters of interstitial fluid are added to the volume of blood the veins already have to carry, this overload of work will weaken the venous system and lead to circulatory disorders. The veins dilate, collecting blood and becoming twisted and enlarged (varicose veins). Sensations of heaviness and pain can be felt in the legs as well.

DISEASES OF IMMUNE DEFICIENCY

There are myriad diseases of immune deficiency. In fact, we can say that all the infectious diseases and those triggered by poisons find a foothold in the body due to immune deficiency.

Adenopathy (Swelling of the Nodes)

One of the best-known diseases of the lymphatic system is the swelling of the nodes, or adenopathy (*adeno* in Greek means "node"). This swelling is caused by the defensive reaction of the node to microbes brought there by the lymph or present in a node where there is an acute infection.

The defensive reaction consists of killing the microbes with the macrophages and lymphocytes it has at its disposal as well as producing lymphocytes that specialize in destroying the problematic microbes. These lymphocytes are manufactured in an extremely high quantity.

The presence of numerous lymphocytes in the node that manufactured them has the inevitable consequence of making it swell. With its tissues congested it becomes hard, and because it is inflamed it is sensitive to the touch. It is easy to feel these kinds of nodes when they are on the surface—for example, at the top of the throat beneath the jawbone during throat or nose infections; in the armpits when suffering from infection in the arms; or in the groin when dealing with infections affecting the legs or lower abdomen.

The nodes will remain swollen for as long as the illness lasts and recover their normal size once it has been overcome.

During a localized infection, such as in the throat or an injury to the skin, only a small group of nodes in a very well circumscribed zone of the body become swollen. During a general infection, such as tuberculosis, AIDS, mononucleosis, and so on, nodes in various areas of the body will be swollen at the same time.

? Did You Know?

Although I have mentioned only microbial infections as a possible cause of adenopathy, it can also be created by the presence of toxins, allergens, or cancer cells (metastasis).

The swelling of the nodes is the result of a defensive action, and that is a good thing. Adenomas can be considered less as an illness than as a symptom of disease. The nodes are not ill. The illness is located where the microbes and poisons that triggered the defensive activity are found.

Cancers

Before discussing cancers that can develop in the lymphatic system, we should first talk about the types and genesis of cancers in general. Generally speaking, we use the word *lymphoma* for cancers that develop in the lymphatic tissues and *leukemia* for cancers that manifest in the blood or bone marrow.

Factors that may cause cancer are multiple and complex.

Some external factors include smoking or chewing tobacco, sun overexposure, industrial chemical poisons, ionizing radiation, and asbestos, among other things, possibly even high intake of spicy food.

According to natural medicine, a cell becomes cancerous if it is immersed in a terrain that is overloaded with both body-produced toxins and those from outside, as well as nutritional deficiencies. In this kind of terrain the cells have been weakened by the deficiencies. Already suffocating under the mass of wastes, they are attacked by the toxic substances. The resulting lesions can affect various elements of the cell, such as the genetic material held in the core (DNA).

The chromosomal changes that result encourage cells to mutate and become cancerous. Cancer cells are abnormal cells that have the distinctive feature of multiplying rapidly, thereby forming a cluster known as a tumor. The proliferation of cancer cells is described as anarchic, or disorderly, because these cells no longer respect the boundaries of the organ to which they belong and begin to invade surrounding tissues. Furthermore, some cells of the tumor can spread into tissues some distance away. When they attach themselves there and multiply, they form a new tumor (metastasis).

It is easy to understand how cells belonging to the lungs, the pancreas, and other organs that have nothing to do with the defense system of the body can become cancerous. But how can cells of the lymph node, an organ that is an integral part of the immune system, become cancerous? Isn't the role of the immune system precisely to defend the cells against such possibilities?

The principal reason why such a thing is possible is that the lymph nodes, like any other organ, are located in the terrain. The cells that form their tissues are irrigated by the bloodstream and surrounded by interstitial fluid. As such, the nodes are immersed in interstitial fluid. They are, therefore, deeply immersed in the body's cellular terrain.

When the composition of this terrain is good, the cells of the nodes are healthy and work normally. When the opposite conditions apply and the composition of the terrain is poor, the cells of the nodes are under attack, and mutations are more likely to take place, which can lead to the development of a tumor.

This is not the whole story, as this harmful influence will be partnered by the inevitable intimate contact of the lymphatic system with toxins, poisons, and various poisonous substances. These substances, after entering the body via the digestive tract or respiratory system, find their way into the interstitial fluid. Their contact with the cells bathed in this fluid constitutes a real danger to these cells. To prevent damage being done to the cells, the lymphatic capillaries—whose role this is—take the burden of these poisons at the same time it absorbs the interstitial fluid. Therefore, the lymphatic system cannot avoid making contact with a significant quantity of the poisons and wastes that enter the body.

The lymph nodes have even closer contact with these undesirable substances because they not only pass them along, as is the case for the lymphatic vessels, but they also hold on to them and confront them in order to destroy them. In other words, the nodes are the battlefield in this battle against poisons and are, therefore, in prolonged contact with them. When circumstances are unfavorable they will take on damage. However, the nodes are not the only organs that can be stricken by a cancer; the lymphatic capillaries, lymphatic vessels, wall muscles of these vessels, bone marrow, and so on can also be afflicted.

This is the way cancerous tumors develop in the lymphatic system, because of overall terrain deficiencies and the close, prolonged contact of lymphatic cells with the poisons.

The form and location of these cancers can be quite varied, so I shall mention only a few.

Hodgkin's Lymphoma

This cancer of the lymph nodes is characterized by changes in the type B lymphocytes. The altered cells multiply to form a tumor.

Non-Hodgkin's Lymphoma

There are a number of types of non-Hodgkin's lymphoma. As a general rule they are characterized by an abnormal elevation of the number of B or T lymphocytes. This multiplication of cells forms a tumor in the lymph node.

Leukemia

The starting point for this disease is the bone marrow, which, as we have seen, produces different kinds of white blood cells that are directly operational as well as lymphocytes that only become active after they have gone through a maturation process in other lymphatic organs.

When the disease is triggered, the bone marrow begins producing a very high number of these cells. They invade the bloodstream and profoundly alter its composition, which stops the body from functioning normally.

Metastatic Tumors

In the cancers described above the proliferation of cells concerned the lymphatic cells, but non-lymphatic cells from separate organs can also develop in the lymphatic system and create tumors.

Normally a proliferation of cancer cells forms a tumor located in the organ to which the cells belong. Some cancerous cells can, however, split off from the tumor and enter the interstitial fluid that surrounds the tumor. From there, due to their large size, they enter the lymphatic system rather than the bloodstream, as the lymphatic capillaries have larger openings than those of the blood capillaries.

When the immune system is strong these mobile cancerous cells are destroyed by the lymphocytes they encounter. However, when the immune system is too weak, these cancer cells are more likely to survive. Instead of being destroyed by the lymphocytes present in the lymph and nodes, they remain alive and active, sometimes taking root in a part of the lymphatic system, such as on the wall of a lymphatic vessel or in a lymph node. When they multiply, these cells form a tumor. It should be pointed out that the characteristics of these tumors are different from those of the lymphatic system. Because they come from another organ, such as the liver or lungs, the tumor is constructed from hepatic, pulmonary, or other cells (and not lymphatic cells).

The problems caused by the development of these tumors are nevertheless similar to those of any tumor: congestion of nearby tissues and organs and the invasion of their tissues by the tumor.

Vulnerability to Infections

When the lymphatic system is weakened, the nodes, spleen, and so on will produce fewer lymphocytes, and these will be of poorer quality. Furthermore, when lymph circulation is slow, lymphocytes are slow to reach the tissues where they are needed to fight an infection, and they arrive in too small a number.

The weakened defensive capabilities of the body allow invaders to easily get the upper hand. The weakening of the lymphatic system therefore leads to greater vulnerability to infection.

Poor functioning of the lymphatic system begins with the accumulation of toxins in the terrain. This creates an environment very favorable to microbes, and they find it easy to settle and multiply there. In this situation microbial infections are able to develop easily and often. "That person catches every passing germ" is the way such people are often described. Colds, laryngitis, flu, or herpes can all ensue. Some people will be affected by only one of these infections, but repeatedly—for example, continuous outbreaks of herpes. Other individuals will be affected sometimes by this disease and sometimes by that one. But this heightened vulnerability also permits infections, such as chronic bronchitis or candida, to install themselves for a long-term stay.

The vulnerability of the body is not only to germs. The immune system acts against everything that it identifies as foreign to the body, including the cancer cells we just discussed as well as allergens. A deficiency in the lymphatic system therefore leads to a weakness of the body's defenses when facing developing tumors and also when dealing with food, respiratory, and skin allergies.

✛ Tips and Tricks

A drop in the body's defensive capacity creates an opportunity for disease, so it's important to keep the immune systems as effective as possible. The major part of the immune system is the lymphatic system, and it is here that therapeutic efforts should be directed.

ILLNESSES CAUSED BY WEAKNESSES IN THE BODY'S DETOXIFYING CAPABILITIES

Natural medicine believes that the overload of the terrain with toxins is the starting point for all diseases (with the exception of those caused by deficiencies). One of the reasons for this toxic overload resides in the weakness of the detoxifying abilities of the lymphatic system.

Lymph transports toxins of a different kind from those carried by the bloodstream. They are larger: large molecules of fat, residue of poorly broken-down starches, cell fragments, dead cells, microbes, and so forth. In natural medicine this detritus is called colloidal waste. It is different from crystalline wastes, or crystals, which are preferably transported by the bloodstream as they are smaller: uric acid, urea, creatinine, pyruvic acid, lactic acid, exhausted minerals, and so forth.

The wastes transported by lymph are partially changed constitutionally before they enter the bloodstream at the subclavian veins. The nodes they need to travel through contain macrophages that swallow and digest them. The noxious substances are transformed this way into smaller and less dangerous, less aggressive wastes.

Just as the proper functioning of the lymphatic system allows effective elimination of toxins, the reverse is true when these abilities are deficient. When toxins collect in the interstitial compartment and in the lymphatic system there are detrimental consequences, as a terrain overloaded with toxins creates a harmful living environment for the cells. Obstructed from functioning properly and injured by aggressive toxins, the cells fall ill, just like the organs they form.

The role of the terrain is therefore paramount. The patient's or therapist's attention is more often focused on the surface by the patient's symptoms and not deeper into the terrain. The symptoms of disease, however, clearly show the profound nature of the problem, for each expresses in its own way the efforts the body makes to eliminate the toxins responsible for the disease.

Skin disorders are caused either by the expulsion of acidic wastes by the sweat-producing glands (for example, dry eczema, cracked skin) or by that of colloidal wastes by the sebaceous glands (such as acne, boils, and weeping eczema).

Cardiovascular diseases have their origin in the presence of colloidal wastes (cholesterol, fatty acids) that thicken the blood, form deposits on the vessels (arteriosclerosis), inflame their walls (phlebitis, arteritis), deform them (varicose veins, hemorrhoids), and clog them (heart attack, stroke, embolism).

People suffering from respiratory ailments blow their noses, cough, or expectorate to rid themselves of colloidal substances clogging their noses (colds), sinuses (sinusitis), throats (sore throat, pharyngitis), bronchia (coughs, bronchitis), or alveoli (asthma).

As brilliantly summarized by the seventeenth-century English physician Thomas Sydenham, nicknamed the English Hippocrates: "A disease, in my opinion, however prejudicial so ever it causes may be to the body, is no more than a vigorous effort of Nature to throw off the morbific matter [toxins], and thus recover the patient." In other words, to cure the patient and keep him alive, the body works with all its strength to eliminate toxins. And one of the great actors in this detoxification is the lymphatic system.

Good to Know

The classification of diseases as acute, chronic, and degenerative testifies to the eliminatory nature of illnesses and the intensity with which the body gets rid of them.

Acute Maladies

In general, acute illnesses can be described as violent and spectacular. The fever accompanying them reveals the intense activity deployed by the body to rid itself of toxins. This activity is expanded to the entire body and all its excretory organs. Flu, for example, is characterized by catarrh (mucous membrane inflammation causing excessive secretion) of the respiratory tract, intestinal disturbances, profuse sweating, and dark urine. Acute illnesses are of short duration because the detoxification efforts are intense and lead to a rapid cleansing of the terrain.

Chronic Diseases

When, over time, excess toxins become too great, the body no longer has enough strength to quickly eliminate toxins that are burdening the terrain, as is the case with acute disease. The body continues striving to eliminate them, but, as its efforts are less intense, it has to repeat them over time; hence, the chronic nature of the disease. The body concentrates its efforts on one organ rather than several. This is why we see a case of bronchitis, an intestinal disorder, or an outbreak of eczema every few months or even weeks. The elimination of toxins is never completed and therefore is attempted repeatedly.

Chronic diseases are, therefore, not general and strong but instead localized and of weak intensity.

Degenerative Diseases

In acute and chronic disease, the body still has sufficient strength to expel its wastes, more or less energetically. In the stage of degenerative illness, this possibility has been lost as the body lacks the necessary strength. Toxins are not expelled properly. The centripetal movement that had prevailed until this point is replaced by a centrifugal movement. Toxins accumulate more and more in the terrain. Cellular life deviates gradually from its normal course, and the living matter becomes increasingly disorganized. This is evidenced by the destruction of certain tissues or organs (sclerosis, irreversible lesions, deformations), the appearance of aberrational compartments in certain cells (cancer cells), or the body's inability to defend itself as an organized entity against microbial invaders (various immune deficiency disorders, AIDS).

The detoxifying capabilities of the lymphatic system therefore play an essential role in ensuring that the body stays healthy. Not only does the lymphatic system rid the terrain of toxins by transporting them to the excretory organs, but it also helps to neutralize them. Any deficiency at this level will compromise overall health. Minor deficiencies will lead to minor disorders, large deficiencies to major diseases.

🎓 What We've Learned

Diseases of the lymphatic system affect its three major functions:

- Circulatory diseases: heavy leg syndrome, swollen ankles, lymphedema, vein problems, cellulitis, weight gain
- Immune deficiency disorders: defensive shortcomings, vulnerability to infections, cancer, leukemia, allergies, and so on
- Illnesses caused by weaknesses in the detoxifying capabilities: toxic overload of the terrain, thickened blood, cardiovascular diseases, rheumatism, eczema, sinusitis, bronchitis, and so on

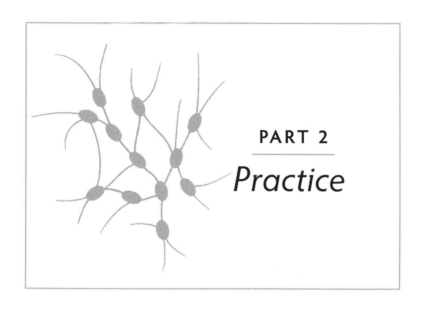

PART 2

Practice

✳ ✳ ✳

There are many therapies that can help to restore the lymphatic system's proper functioning. Each therapy on its own is helpful, but some are more so because they work more directly on the source of the problem. A hierarchy of remedies will help to avoid the situation in which an individual uses secondary and less effective remedies. This is why I have classified these therapies into three major groups: general therapies, special therapies, and complementary therapies.

GENERAL THERAPIES

We could also call general therapies the foundational therapies, as they attack the primary causes of the lymphatic system's weakness. For this reason, they are recommended for everyone:

- Changing your diet (chapter 7)
- Draining toxins via the excretory organs (chapter 8)
- Physical exercise (chapter 9)
- Hydration (chapter 10)

SPECIAL THERAPIES

Special therapies aim at stimulating the lymphatic system in a specific manner. Because they do not address the profound causes for its weakened state, they cannot bring about a cure on their own. However, they are very helpful when used in combination with a foundational therapy:

- Medicinal plants (chapter 11)
- Rapid detoxification through diet (chapter 12)
- Dry diet and dry fasting (chapter 13)

- Lymphatic drainage massage (chapter 14)
- Foot reflexology (chapter 15)

COMPLEMENTARY THERAPIES

Complementary therapies are useful supplements to the general treatments but of lesser importance than the special therapies, as their effect on the lymphatic system is not as powerful:

- Deep, full breathing (chapter 16)
- Trampoline (chapter 17)
- Compression therapy (chapter 18)

Each therapy noted here has its own chapter explaining its objectives and the means to put it into practice. All twelve therapies should not be implemented. While the foundational therapies are for everyone, choose only one or two of the others based on your personal needs. For example, follow a detoxifying diet if your terrain is overly saturated with toxins; do foot reflexology if the lymphatic vessels are lazy and need to be stimulated; use a trampoline if physical exercise is not possible, and so forth.

Another way to proceed is to top off the basic treatments by successively doing a one-month cure with each of the special therapies—for instance, one month of draining, one month of medicinal plants, and so on.

✪ Tips and Tricks

Some techniques will turn out to be better for you than others, and these are the ones you will need to use to continue your treatment.

7

Changing Your Diet

The cleaner the fluid, the easier it will flow. Because it is less viscous, it circulates with greater ease. Conversely, when liquid is thick and heavy, its movement is more difficult. This is true for all the bodily fluids, including lymph. When it loses its fluidity because it has to transport too many toxins, it circulates slowly and allows the toxins to start collecting in the terrain.

Most toxins originate in the food we eat. There are other ways that toxins can get into the body, such as the lungs and skin, but food remains their largest source.

The ability of food to contribute toxins varies from one kind of food to the next. For this reason a distinction is made between two major types of food: heavy foods, which are the source of many toxins, and light foods, whose use by the body yields very few toxins.

HEAVY FOODS

Heavy foods are the ones that are concentrated. They contain little water but a great deal of solid material. This material includes complex substances—fats, starches, and proteins—all of which require quite a bit of work to be digested and metabolized. They are the source of numerous toxins.

Examples of heavy foods include:

Fats	Heat-pressed oils, cold cuts, sausages, hydrogenated margarine, fried foods, chips, pastries
Animal flesh	Red meat, fowl, fish, shellfish, seafood
Dairy products	Hard and soft cheeses, cream, butter
Grains	Wheat, rice, rye, oats
Grain by-products	Flour, bread, pasta, crackers, cookies, cold cereal flakes, some snack chips
Legumes	Lentils, soy beans, peas, green beans, white beans, fava beans
White sugar	Chocolate, cake, ice cream, candy, jam, soda, desserts in general
Drinks	Coffee, tea, chocolate, alcohol

LIGHT FOODS

Light foods are not very concentrated and have a high water content. They primarily contain fiber, vitamins, minerals, and trace elements. When consumed they create very few toxins.

Examples of light foods include:

Fresh fruits	Apples, pears, plums, apricots, oranges, tangerines, grapefruits
Small fruits	Strawberries, raspberries, blueberries, cherries, blackberries, red and black currants
Dried fruits	Raisins, prunes, dried apricots, figs, dates
Fruit juices	Apple, orange, grape (without added sugar)
Leafy vegetables	Salad greens, kale, spinach, cabbage
Stalk vegetables	Beet greens, celery, leeks, asparagus

Root vegetables	Carrots, celery root, kohlrabi, turnip, radish
Vegetable fruits	Tomato, pepper, zucchini, squash, cucumber
Vegetable flowers	Cauliflower, broccoli, brussels sprouts, artichoke
Vegetable juices	Carrot, beet
Starches	Potatoes, chestnuts
Oleaginous fruits	Almonds, hazelnuts, walnuts, olives
Seeds	Sunflower, sesame, pumpkin, chia
Dairy products	Cottage cheese, plain (unsweetened) yogurt

THE PRIMARY CAUSES OF THICKENING OF THE LYMPH BY FOOD TOXINS

Mistaken food choices are frequently the source of toxin overload in the terrain and in the lymph. Following are the most common errors.

Overconsumption of Fats

A large portion of the fats from the digestion process are transported by the lymph. This is especially true for large fat molecules, meaning those high in saturated fatty acids. These primarily come from fatty substances prepared specifically for human consumption: heat-pressed oil, hydrogenated margarine, shortening, and butter.

Overconsumption of fats occurs when you cook with a significant amount of butter, hydrogenated margarine, oil, or cream. Foods that are harmful in this category include fried foods, rich cream sauces, chips, and pastries.

Overconsumption of Proteins

Even just a century ago, consumption of meat, fish, and cheese was rather modest because these products were rare and expensive. Today the reverse is true. Consumption of these foods has become quite commonplace. They often represent the largest part of the meal, whereas because of their concentrated nature, they should be the smallest.

Overconsumption of proteins occurs when you eat more than about 200 grams (7 ounces) of meat at a single meal, meat or fish every day, or meat twice a day. Or when you eat a meal that has several different forms of protein such as a fish appetizer, a meat entrée, and cheese for dessert. The National Academy of Medicine recommends a daily protein intake of 0.8 gram per each kilo of body weight. A simple formula for determining the body's daily protein needs in grams is to multiply your weight in pounds by 0.36.

Cheese is a protein that is also high in saturated fat, so it should not be eaten in too large a quantity.

Too many leguminous proteins can also produce a lot of colloidal wastes.

Overconsumption of Starch

While some people eat too many proteins or fats, others eat excessive amounts of flour-based foods, such as bread, pasta, cereal flakes, or rice.

The excess of flour-based foods can take place over the course of a single meal or because each meal of the day contains a flour product: toast, cereal, or a pastry at breakfast; rice at noon; bread and pasta in the evening; and perhaps cookies for a snack.

Overconsumption of White Sugar

Average consumption of added sugar in the industrialized world is about 100 grams (7 tablespoons) a day. This includes sugar added to various beverages (coffee, tea, and so on) as well as the sugar found in many foods: soda, cookies, jam, pastries, desserts, and even bread, ketchup, and some seasonings.

General Overeating

General overconsumption is taking place when someone combines many or all of the different kinds of overconsumed foods noted above, eating excessive amounts of fats, proteins, starches, and sugars.

Overeating of any kind inevitably leads to toxic overload. The larger the excesses, the higher the quantity of toxins that will be produced. The toxin overload can come with or without weight gain.

Any individual suffering from a weakened lymphatic system or suffering from diseases affecting this system has a terrain overloaded with toxins and needs dietary reform. Such a reform is also indicated for those who have been eating poorly and wish to prevent future disorder of this organ system.

Because the diet that is detrimental for the lymphatic system is characterized by the excess of bad fats, proteins, starches, and white sugar, consumption of these foods must be reduced. Reduction does not mean elimination, as these are basic foods (with the exception of the bad fats and white sugar) that the body needs. Not eating *any* of them will cause deficiencies that can lead to illness.

The typical diet (sometimes called SAD, or standard American diet) consists of 70 percent heavy foods and 30 percent light foods. This can easily be seen on the plate of the average meal. Three-quarters of the plate is occupied by meat and starch (pasta, potatoes, or rice) and the other quarter by vegetables. In a healthy diet these proportions are reversed. Light foods should represent 70 percent of the meal and heavy foods 30 percent. (The percentages indicated here are meant to serve as an illustration and should not be taken literally or used to calculate and weigh food rations.)

✛ Tips and Tricks

One cause of overeating is snacking. Some people eat constantly between meals. All these little snacks add up to a large quantity of food that overloads the body with toxins and tires the digestive system.

IMPLEMENTING A REFORMED DIET

A reformed diet will concretely lead to a diet that is natural, healthy, and low in toxins. The small quantities of toxins generated by this kind of diet will be easily eliminated by the body.

The following example is based on current Western dietary norms. The purpose is to give a general idea of the way we can eat but should of course be adjusted to reflect your personal situation. Whether you have a physically demanding or sedentary job, stressful or not, or a large and demanding family, or if you have trouble metabolizing certain foods, the proportion of foods appearing in the diet can vary—for example, fewer fatty foods for people with weak livers, more starch and protein for those who are more physically active, more vegetables and whole grains for the person who needs fiber to mitigate constipation, and so forth.

The quality of the foods is also important, of course. You should give preference to whole foods: brown rice, whole-grain bread, whole-grain pasta. These foods still contain all their valuable vitamins, minerals, and trace elements, unlike refined foods, from which they have been removed. Heat-pressed oils will be eschewed in favor of cold-pressed virgin oils, and whole unprocessed sugar will replace refined white sugar. Whenever possible, priority should be given to foods grown organically.

Sample Menu
(to be adjusted to personal needs and tastes)

Breakfast	
Herbal tea	Mint, verbena, thyme, ginger, or rosemary
Dark bread	Whole grain, pumpernickel, or brown bread
	+ butter or plant-based margarine high in unsaturated fatty acids
	+ honey, maple syrup, or low-fat cheese
OR	
Cottage cheese or unsweetened yogurt	
	+ fresh fruit
	+ dried fruit
	+ nuts or seeds
Morning Snack	
Drink	Water, herbal tea (no sugar), fruit juice (no added sugar), or vegetable juice
Your choice	Fresh fruits
	Dried fruits
	Blend of dried fruits and nuts
	Whole-grain cookies

Noon Meal	
Drink	Water, herbal tea (no sugar), or vegetable juice
Green salad or crudités	
	+ cooked vegetables or homemade vegetable soup
	+ one protein: cheese, eggs, fish, or meat
	+ a low-fat starch: potatoes, pasta, or brown rice
Afternoon Snack	
Drink	Water, herbal tea (no sugar), fruit juice (sugar free), or vegetable juice
Your choice	Fresh fruits or dried fruits
	Whole-grain crackers with cheese or a little almond/peanut butter
	Yogurt or kefir
Evening Meal	
Drink	Water, unsweetened herbal tea, or vegetable juice
Green salad or crudités	
	+ cooked vegetables or homemade vegetable soup
	+ one protein: cheese, eggs, fish, or meat
	+ a low-fat starch: potatoes, pasta, or brown rice

Initially, changing your diet will require some effort to get organized and several days or weeks to get used to the new composition of your meals. These efforts will be rewarded quickly, however, as digestion becomes easier and you will feel better and have more energy. With regard to your cellular terrain, there will be a sharp reduction of toxins, which will help your lymphatic system as well as the rest of your body.

🎓 What We've Learned

- An overload of toxins is the origin of most diseases.
- The primary source of toxins is food.
- Changing your diet is essential. The goal is to reduce the amount of foods you eat that produce a lot of toxins and increase the amount of those that produce few toxins.

8

Stimulating the Excretory Organs

Because the accumulation of toxins in the cellular terrain is the starting point for the majority of diseases, people suffering from ailments affecting the lymphatic system usually have a terrain that is overburdened by wastes. They typically have an even larger quantity, because the lymphatic system is an organ for eliminating them. When the system is weakened or ill, many toxins will not be eliminated and end up collecting inside this system.

☝ Good to Know

Natural medicine treats the accumulation of disease-causing toxins with a therapy intended to detoxify the body; in other words, freeing the terrain of the overloads burdening it. We call this effort draining the toxins.

Toxins cannot just leave the body wherever they please but must pass through assigned exits—the excretory organs. There are five of these organs: the liver, intestines, kidneys, skin, and lungs. There are no other exits for toxins, which means we have to concentrate our efforts on them to detoxify the body.

The function of the excretory organs is to rid the body of toxins. Many people believe this work takes place automatically and under any and all circumstances, but just like any other organ, the excretory organs can also be saturated with toxins; in other words, toxins that have collected in their tissues can prevent them from functioning properly. In such cases they are less capable of filtering and eliminating wastes. The exit doors are only partially open. In everyday language we say these organs are "closed" and that we have to "open" them in order to restart eliminating toxins properly.

THE CRITERIA FOR GOOD AND BAD EXCRETORY ORGAN FUNCTIONING

What criteria must the various excretory organs meet to be considered open? The signs of good and bad functioning I describe below should give the reader a good idea of how well or poorly his or her emunctory organs are working.

The Liver

When the liver is functioning correctly digestion takes place easily and well. When the opposite is true the following disorders appear:

- Frequent attacks of indigestion
- Difficulty digesting fats: heavy meals, some meats, eggs, cream, cheese
- Nausea
- Bloating, belching
- Fatigue and a feeling of heaviness after meals

- Dry or pasty mouth, white or furry tongue
- Migraine, headaches after meals
- Sallow complexion

The Intestines

Good intestinal functioning is revealed by:

- Daily evacuation (even twice a day); stools are eliminated easily and thoroughly.
- An intestinal transit of twenty-four to thirty-six hours.

☝ Good to Know

The speed of the intestinal transit is an important element to monitor; wastes should leave our bodies in the form of stools about twenty-four hours after ingestion; this means that every day we should evacuate what we ate the preceding day. We can evacuate stools every twenty-four hours without necessarily having a twenty-four-hour transit. In some of these cases matter accumulates in the intestines and new arrivals push what accumulated the day or days before into the bottom of the digestive tract so that stools appear to be eliminated every day, but in reality there is a three- or four-day delay.

- Stools should be a light-brown color.
- They should have a pasty and solid consistency, thus neither hard and dry nor too liquid.
- There should be minimal intestinal gas. The too-frequent or even habitual presence of gas (bloating)

is a sign that transit is too slow and foods are fermenting or putrefying.

The Kidneys

Good kidney function can be recognized when it meets the following criteria:

- The volume of urine eliminated daily rises to approximately 1.5 liters, the volume required to adequately transport toxins out of the body.
- The number of daily urinations is at least five, as the need to urinate makes itself felt when the bladder content reaches aboout 3 deciliters.
- The color of urine is normally lemon yellow; when it is colorless or pale the kidneys are not eliminating enough wastes. However, in people who drink a lot of fluids over the course of the day, the absence of color is normal, as the large amounts of liquid they consume dilute the urine.
- Everyone recognizes the smell of urine, but it can be missing in cases of renal laziness because the kidneys are eliminating fewer toxins.

The Skin

The skin has two kinds of glands for eliminating toxins: sweat-producing glands and sebaceous glands.

Sweat glands evacuate wastes in perspiration. The signs they are functioning properly include:

- The skin sweats. In other words, it becomes moist or clammy when the environment is hot or the individual is making a physical effort.

- Perspiration occurs all over and is not limited to small surfaces such as the armpits, feet, or head.
- The odor of sweat is usually pleasant or neutral; if it is malodorous it is charged with toxins, which is not a bad sign in itself as toxins are being expelled from the body, but it does indicate that there are a lot of them and they have not been properly eliminated until now.
- The absence of pimples, dry eczema, and hives. These disorders appear only when toxins are causing congestion in the sweat glands.

The sebaceous glands eliminate toxins in an oily secretion—sebum. In addition to its role as an eliminator, sebum also lubricates the skin, so when the skin is dry it indicates that these glands are not working well. When the sebaceous glands are working well the skin

- is supple, as it is well lubricated by the sebum; and
- has no pimples (acne) or weeping eczema.

The Lungs

Signs that the respiratory tract is working well are the following:

- The nasal passages are unclogged, and air enters them freely and easily.
- The need to blow your nose is rare and usually occurs to get rid of dust.
- There is an absence of phlegm and mucus clogging the nostrils or throat or collecting in the bronchia, thereby creating a need to blow your nose, cough, or expectorate.

- When you jog a little until you're out of breath there is no need to spit and expectorate, a condition that would mean the respiratory tract is encumbered by wastes and is working poorly.

☝ Good to Know

The most important excretory organs for the lymphatic system are the liver, intestines, and sebaceous glands, because they eliminate the colloidal waste that is the main type of waste transported by the lymphatic system.

DRAINING

Draining is a means of eliminating collected toxins that have made the body sick.

A draining consists of stimulating the elimination work of the excretory organs. The types of drainers are varied and range from medicinal plants and juices or foods with detoxifying properties to massage, colon cleanse, sauna, and so on.

The excretory organs are the essential avenue for draining. This is why in a draining cure all efforts are focused on them with the goal of restoring normal elimination. Or, even better, it will increase this elimination over a certain period of time in order to make up for the delay.

First of all, it is the excretory organ itself that, stimulated by the drainers, will purify itself of the wastes stagnating inside and clogging its filter. Once the excretory organ has been cleansed it will once again be capable of filtering blood properly. When the bloodstream has been rid of its toxins it is better able to take charge of those collected in the deep tissues, including the interstitial fluid, so it can then carry them to the excretory organs. With the resulting cleansing of the interstitial fluid, the lymph will be less burdened with wastes and will circulate better, allowing the lymph nodes to gradually get rid of the toxins overloading them.

A draining is therefore characterized by an increase in the quantity of waste produced by the excretory organs. This increased elimination must be visible to the person taking the cure. The matter evacuated by the intestines is more abundant or the evacuations are more regular; urine takes on a darker color because it is charged with more waste, and it will also increase in volume; the skin will sweat more copiously; and the respiratory tract will free itself of the colloidal wastes that are impeding its proper functioning.

Corresponding to this visible evacuation of wastes is a reduction of the toxin content held in the tissues, the interstitial fluid, and the lymph. The terrain becomes clean again, and consequently the person's overall state improves while the disorders that had been present will gradually diminish and disappear. This is true for all the organs, including lymphatic organs such as the nodes and spleen. The healing possibilities are obviously dependent on the scope of the damage already inflicted on the organs by the wastes and the regenerative capabilities of these organs.

Two other important factors that need to be taken into consideration are the effectiveness and duration of the cure.

A draining's effectiveness depends on its intensity. The dose of the drainers, therefore, must be well regulated. It can't be too low as this will not stimulate eliminations sufficiently, and no results will be seen. But it cannot be too high as this will exhaust the body and possibly damage the excretory organs with too large an influx of toxins. The optimum dose is therefore the one that falls between these two extremes.

The optimal dose is different for every individual's body, and there are no mathematical rules to define it. Each body must find its correct dose, starting with small doses that are increased gradually. Starting with large doses and then reducing them is a bad approach, as these large doses disrupt and exhaust the body, making it even more difficult to identify the right dose.

The duration of the cure also plays a fundamental role. The cleansing process produced by the different kinds of draining is a physiological process and shows profound effects only over the long term. The body cannot simply empty itself all at once of toxins it has collected over months if not years. To the contrary, these toxins are removed from the body little by little. To be effective a cure must last over a period of weeks; one or two months would be preferable. Most often, it will need to be repeated several times during the year.

The excretory organs should not be stimulated all at the same time. When a draining is performed for the first time, it is preferable that it initially stimulate only one organ so as to avoid dispersing the body's forces. In this case choose the organ that is most deficient. Later a person can stimulate two or three at the same time.

DRAINING IN PRACTICE

For each excretory organ I provide an example of a medicinal plant and describe the way it should be taken to stimulate the work of filtering and eliminating. This will be primarily mother tinctures (low-potency combinations of a botanical extract with a specific amount of alcohol), but these plants can also be consumed in the form of gel caps, tablets, or infusions. Complementary methods for supporting the drainer's work will also be provided.

The Liver

One of the best plants for draining the liver is dandelion. It is well known because it has been used successfully for centuries.

❦ Dandelion (*Taraxacum*)

Dosage: 20 to 50 drops of a mother tincture (MT) three times a day with water before meals.

Complementary method: Hot water bottle. This is a hollow rubber sac that can be filled with hot water from the tap. Placed on the body over the liver, its heat deeply penetrates this area and greatly intensifies the work of the liver. Apply a hot water bottle over the liver region for a period of thirty minutes once or twice a day. You can do this, for example, after a meal while reading or watching a TV program.

The Intestines

One of the most useful laxative plants is alder buckthorn. It is easily tolerated by everyone as its effect is so gentle.

❦ Alder Buckthorn (*Rhamnus frangula*)

Dosage: 20 to 50 drops of a mother tincture (MT) with water before going to bed. The effect will appear the next morning.

Complementary method: Flaxseed. Thanks to their high mucilage content, these seeds expand five times in contact with water, thereby providing the intestines with a large quantity of roughage. This will greatly facilitate movement in the intestinal transit and elimination of toxins. Take 2–6 teaspoons of flaxseed a day with a large glass of water, all at once or in two helpings.

The Kidneys

Pilosella has a powerful diuretic and disinfecting effect in the urinary tract.

❦ Pilosella (*Pilosella*)

Dosage: 20–50 drops of a mother tincture (MT), three times a day with water before meals.

Complementary method: Water cure. Water consumed in large quantities has a diuretic effect because it forces the kidneys to work harder. Drinking a liter of water more than your usual consumption of fluids stimulates the kidneys to eliminate a lot more toxins. Drink one additional liter of water every day.

The Skin

Some plants encourage the work of the sweat glands. They help the body to sweat, hence their name of sudorific plants. Their active ingredients not only induce sweating but also increase sweating triggered by heat or physical activity.

❦ Elderberry Flowers (*Sambucus nigra*)
or Linden Flowers (*Tilia europaea*)

Dosage: 1 tablespoon of flowers per cup steeped for ten minutes. Drink two or three cups a day while still very hot.

Complementary method: Physical exercise. The body's production of heat clearly increases during physical activity.

The sweat produced by physical activity is more copious and more charged with toxins because cellular exchanges are intensified. You will sweat more if the activity takes place in the sun or if you are wearing an additional layer of clothing that prevents body heat from escaping. Practice your choice of physical activity (jogging, tennis, walking, gardening, bike riding) two or three times a week.

Lungs

Eucalyptus is regularly used for the respiratory tract. It makes the wastes collected in the lungs more fluid, thereby making them easier to eliminate by expectoration.

❧ Eucalyptus (*Eucalyptus globulus*)

Dosage: 1 or 2 capsules (500–750 mg) three times a day with water before meals.

Complementary method: Jogging. A running walk done in a mild, pleasant rhythm, jogging accentuates the movements of inhalation and exhalation, which loosens the wastes of the respiratory tract and helps the body to cough them up, thereby eliminating them.

With the various methods of draining, the body can detoxify itself. Numerous toxins will be eliminated, and the terrain will become cleaner and cleaner. The organs will function better, including those of the lymphatic system. The walls of the lymphatic vessels will recover their tone, which in turn will help lymph circulate more easily. The lymph nodes will work more intensely. In this way they will filter and neutralize many more toxins and microbes.

🎓 What We've Learned

Like all the body's organs, the lymphatic system will become ill if there is an overload of toxins in the terrain. Healing this system breakdown requires cleansing the terrain. This can be achieved by draining the toxins out of the body with the help of medicinal plants. The five organs responsible for the elimination of toxins are the liver, intestines, kidneys, skin, and lungs.

9

Establishing an Exercise Routine

Physical activity has a beneficial effect on the circulation of lymph in two different ways: one is by acting on it indirectly through the intermediary of the blood circulation, and the other is by acting directly on the lymphatic vessels.

INDIRECT EFFECT VIA THE BLOODSTREAM

Physical activity raises the speed of blood circulation, and thereby blood pressure. In this way the bloodstream will then intensify the formation of interstitial fluid and its penetration into the lymphatic capillaries and therefore into the lymphatic system. This is why good blood circulation encourages good lymph circulation.

There are many obstacles to good blood circulation, however. Blood has a certain heaviness that has to be surmounted—for example, when the bloodstream has to ascend back to the heart from the legs. Additionally, blood gets thicker when it is overburdened with toxins. Its viscosity increases, which hinders its progress. Blood capillaries also have an effect on blood circulation due to their slenderness.

Although the arteries and veins have a larger diameter than the capillaries, when toxins become deposited on their walls the ability of blood to pass through them is diminished. These toxin deposits make the walls less supple and flexible, and the rigidity this causes prevents them from properly maintaining blood circulation through rhythmic contraction and dilation. Furthermore, blood crossing through the organs can be compared to a river having to go through a narrow channel—there is a braking effect.

All these obstacles can be avoided or reduced thanks to physical exercise. In fact, physical activity is only possible thanks to repeated contractions of the muscles. The efforts they are making increase their need for oxygen, which impels the lungs to breathe more deeply and rapidly. As this oxygen is carried into the muscles by the bloodstream, its circulation must also accelerate, which forces the heart to pump more energetically. This is how, thanks to physical exercise, the entire blood circulation system is put into service. Its working rhythm intensifies with the happy result of accelerating lymph circulation.

Thanks to this acceleration, lymph leaves the lymphatic system to enter the bloodstream more quickly and carries the toxins along with it. The lymph thereby loses its viscosity and is better able to carry away the toxins that are deposited on the walls of the lymphatic vessels and nodes. Freed of the toxins that had been obstructing them, these organs can once again perform their detoxifying and immune system duties. The benefits that result will be helpful no matter what problems the lymphatic system may be experiencing.

DIRECT EFFECT ON
THE LYMPHATIC VESSELS

To truly realize the direct effect of physical exercise on the lymphatic vessels, we have to remember that the lymphatic system doesn't have a lymphatic heart to pump lymph. Lymph progresses through the vessels thanks to the alternating contractions and dilations of the vessel walls, which apply pressure to this fluid. But these are not the only pressures. There are others that come from external sources: muscle contractions, the movements of breathing, and the pulsing of the blood vessels. All three of these aids to lymph circulation are reinforced by physical exercise.

✚ Tips and Tricks

Ever wonder why doctors and other health care providers keep encouraging you to exercise? Every muscle you are aware of moving has an effect on internal vessel walls, helping your body to move blood where it's needed and move out toxins. Beyond making you strong, exercise also helps to keep you healthy.

Muscle Contractions

During physical efforts, the muscles dilate and compress the surrounding tissues, including the lymphatic capillaries and vessels. Compressed by the muscles, the walls of these channels press strongly on their contents, thereby forcing the lymph to leave its present location for a spot farther along in the vessel. Thanks to the valves in the vessels, the lymph can travel in only one direction—forward toward the thoracic duct, then toward the bloodstream in the area of the subclavian veins. Physical exercises don't cause a single contraction of one muscle but rather repeated contractions of numerous muscles, thus ensuring that large areas of the lymphatic network are stimulated. Thanks to this external support, lymph will circulate much more easily in the stimulated area as well as have a repercussion everywhere else in the lymphatic network.

The Movements of Breathing

Strong pressure is also applied on the lymphatic vessels by the dilation of the lungs during physical activity. The lungs swell prominently and take up a much larger space, which creates the same crushing effect on the surrounding tissues as that caused by muscle contractions. The lymphatic vessels that will be stimulated are those in close proximity to the lungs. These vessels are quite numerous and include among them two large and important ones: the right and left thoracic ducts. The acceleration of lymph circulation at this level will also have beneficial effects farther along in the entire lymphatic system.

? Did You Know?

When resting we take in only about a half liter of air on an inhale; during physical exercise this volume increases to three or four liters.

The Pulsing of the Blood Vessels

Blood vessels are continuously propelled by alternating movements of contraction and dilation that cause their contents to move forward through the vessel. These movements are generated by contractions of the heart and the muscle fibers present in the vessel walls. These pulsations may be quite small, but they trigger the compression of neighboring tissues with every dilation.

As a great many of the lymphatic vessels follow the same paths as those of the blood vessels, the two kinds of vessels are thereby side by side. Consequently, every dilation of the blood vessels compresses the neighboring lymphatic vessels, pushing forward the lymph they contain. Because these pulsing movements take place continually, lymphatic circulation is permanently sustained by the circulatory system. This support can be reinforced by physical exercise. The activity accelerates the scope of the pulsations and their rhythm and consequently the scope of the pressure applied to the lymphatic vessels.

🖐 Good to Know

The acceleration of lymphatic circulation through exercise is real and measurable. When a person is resting, lymph circulates through the thoracic duct at a rate of 100 milliliters (just under 3.5 ounces) an hour. Depending on the intensity of the physical exercise, the flow can reach 1,000 to 3,000 ml; in other words, ten to thirty times greater.

THE PRACTICE OF PHYSICAL EXERCISE

The ability to do physical exercise when suffering from illnesses of the lymphatic system varies from one person to the next.

Someone suffering from problems concerning the immune system and detoxification functions is generally capable of performing most physical activities and therefore has many options. Conversely, when a disorder is affecting the circulatory system, which is exhibited by the formation of lymphedemas, choices are more limited. For someone suffering from lymphedema, an overly intense physical activity could exacerbate the problems rather than improve them. Such a person should perform only special exercises adjusted to ability, with the goal of decongesting the affected limbs.

Physical Activity for People with No Restrictions on Mobility

To have any effect, physical activity must be sufficiently intense to overcome fluids' force of inertia and accelerate blood circulation, and thereby that of lymph. A quiet stroll will not cause profound acceleration unless it goes for at least twenty to thirty minutes. But all it takes is an intense effort for two to three minutes—a sprint on a bike, for example—for circulation to spike, causing a subsequent acceleration of lymph circulation. Getting winded is a sign that circulation is accelerated, because the two things go hand in hand.

However, the goal is not to rapidly raise the speed of the blood's circulation and cause it to spike sharply, only to abandon it shortly afterward because exhaustion prevents continuation of the effort. That effect on the lymph will be minimal, because the acceleration was only temporary. Rather, the objective is to perform a physical activity long enough—a good hour or more—that acceleration of the bloodstream will last over a long period. This is the only way lymph circulation will also pick up speed, permitting some of the toxin-saturated lymph to be eliminated and replaced with clean lymph.

What Kinds of Physical Activities?

All forms of physical activity are an option here because it all has a beneficial effect on circulation. Choosing ones you enjoy doing will make it easier to spend time doing them regularly and for long-enough periods of time to get results.

Here are a few examples of physical activities, but this list is far from exhaustive: walking, jogging, biking, dancing, swimming, rowing, various gymnastics, team games (soccer, volleyball, basketball), skiing, skating, gardening, and so forth.

Frequency

Lymphatic circulation accelerates only during the time you perform a physical activity and for a short time afterward and then resumes its normal rhythm. It is preferable to not allow too much time to elapse between sessions. The ideal is to do some kind of physical activity every day. In this way the lymphatic system will be stimulated repeatedly. It will not have time to fall back asleep and its movement will be reengaged every time you exert yourself physically for a good half hour or so. (You want to feel your core temperature rise and sustain that for at least twenty minutes.)

If a daily session is not possible, it's important to stick to a schedule of every two or three days. However, to keep the lymphatic system from slowing down too much during the days off, it's a good idea to arrange things that will nonetheless place demands on it. A lack of time is often cited as an argument against daily exercise, and indeed, going to a fitness club, tennis court, dance venue, and so on takes time. One solution to this problem is to introduce more movement into your daily life so that it can merge into what you do every day. For example, take the stairs rather than an elevator; get off the bus one stop before your regular stop and maneuver the last leg of your journey on foot; ride a bicycle to your destination whenever possible. Or go right out the front door and jog or walk around the area for twenty minutes.

There are endless ways of being more physical and thereby stimulating lymphatic circulation, especially if we don't limit ourselves to just one but instead incorporate several into our lives.

Gradual Progression

For people who have not been very physically active previously, it is recommended to introduce these exercise sessions into your life gently so the body can gradually get accustomed to them.

✚ Tips and Tricks

It makes sense to schedule exercise sessions in advance and clearly determine the days and hours when they can take place. If we simply tell ourselves, "I will do a session every day when I have the time", there is a high risk of sessions not happening.

Implementation

In the beginning it takes effort to get organized and establish a rhythm, but over time physical exercise becomes a habit. It's a pleasure to spend time this way, and when you have to skip a session, you will feel like you are missing out on something.

Physical Activities for People with Limited Range of Movement

People suffering from lymphedema are restricted in their movements. Their legs or arms have become swollen and cannot move easily.

What Physical Activities Are Possible for Limited Range?

Intense physical activities are to be avoided, because they can cause more harm than good. For example, when great demands are put on the leg muscles, blood circulation speeds up in this region. The raised blood pressure increases the formation of interstitial fluid, which is removed by the lymphatic system. But if this system has been weakened by lymphedema, it is incapable of eliminating the excess interstitial fluid. It then stagnates in the tissues and combines with what is already there, which increases the size of the lymphedema.

This does not mean that people suffering from lymphedemas are condemned to immobility. Movement will do them much good, but it has to be adjusted to the specific situation. It will then be very beneficial, as it encourages decongestion of the edemas.

A specially perfected system for lymphedema sufferers is the Casley-Smith method, a complex physical therapy that combines breathing, movement, compression, and massage. It is taught by specialists, but once learned, the exercises can be practiced solo at home.

🎓 What We've Learned

Physical exercise stimulates the lymphatic system in two ways:

- Increased circulation of the blood accelerates the circulation of lymph.
- Muscle contraction, dilation of the lungs, and pulsation of blood vessels exert repeated pressure on the lymphatic vessels, which pushes the lymph forward.

10

Improving Hydration

Good hydration of the body is essential for the survival and proper functioning of cells. Cells entirely depend on body fluids for oxygenation, food, and the removal of toxins. A sufficient quantity of liquid must be provided continually. The lymphatic system is particularly dependent on intake of liquid.

In fact, the water we drink travels through the intestinal walls to enter the blood vessels and maintain blood volume. It is only when this volume is of sufficient size that the plasma (serum) leaves the blood capillaries to enter the interstitial milieu. Once it is there, the plasma—now called interstitial fluid—can enter the lymphatic capillaries to become lymph. This latter, therefore, holds third position in the general circulation of fluids, after blood and interstitial fluid.

Negative repercussions on lymph occur when the body is not taking in enough liquids. Given the fact that this means a reduction of blood volume, it can no longer yield enough of the fluid required by the interstitial compartment. The resulting lower volume of interstitial fluid that flows out reduces the potential for lymph formation. This means that the lymph will be more viscous, and circulation will be sluggish.

The body must therefore receive enough water on a daily

basis to function properly. But what exactly is sufficient? How much liquid does this imply?

The answers to these questions can be found by measuring the volume of water lost by the human body every day. The amount of water lost is the amount that needs to be replaced. We will look at those quantities in the next section.

WATER'S WAYS OF LEAVING THE BODY

Four exit paths are used for fluid to leave our bodies. It should come as no surprise that these four exits are excretory organs.

The Kidneys

The kidneys form the principal excretory organ for eliminating fluids. Every day we eliminate approximately 1.5 liters of water in the form of urine, which is actually 95 percent water and 5 percent solid materials.

The Skin

Water exits the skin through perspiration or transpiration. Perspiration is an excretion of urea, uric acids, and some salts that takes place continuously. It is mostly invisible to the naked eye, as the little drops of sweat that reach the skin's surface evaporate immediately.

Transpiration is episodic, occurs in greater quantity than with perspiration, and the sweat droplets are larger, which means they are visible. This happens during physical exertion or when the external temperature is very hot.

On average, the body sweats 0.8 liter a day. This volume can climb to 2 to 3 liters during intense physical effort, fever, or a sauna.

The Lungs

In a breath exhalation, a certain amount of liquid leaves the body in the form of vapor. This eliminates about 0.4 liter of water a day. The rate is higher when doing exercise or playing sports.

The Intestines

The intestines are the excretory organ that eliminates the smallest quantity of water. Although the 150 grams (about 5 ounces) of stool we eliminate every day look solid, their liquid content is about 120 grams. This liquid is necessary to ensure smooth evacuation.

The total amount of water eliminated daily by these four organs is 2.5 liters, or close to 3 quarts. This is consequently the volume of liquid that needs to be replaced in the body every day to cover its fluid needs.

The body receives this liquid from beverages as well as from food, particularly fruits and vegetables with a water content that can be up to 95 percent of their weight. Some people's water needs are covered primarily by the water contained in the foods they eat and secondarily by drinks; for others it is the opposite.

✚ Tips and Tricks

According to different studies, and taking modern lifestyle into consideration—individual stress, overheated buildings, a diet that may be rich in salt and sugar but poor in fruits and vegetables—daily consumption of water should be about 2.5 liters (or ten 8-ounce glasses). This will vary depending on body size, age, activity level, climate, and so on.

THE PRACTICE OF HYDRATION

For most people, daily fluid intake needs to be a focused effort, especially for those just starting to pay attention. Eventually it can become habitual.

Measuring Your Daily Consumption

To determine your personal liquid consumption, measure throughout the day the volume of every drink you consume. The intake can vary from one day to the next. It is good to take these measurements for three or four days in a row.

With the help of a calibrated container, measure the volume of water for the glass you use regularly. After this, you need only note this volume every time you consume a drink using this glass or cup.

Every day, calculate the total volume of liquid intake in the form of water, herbal tea, and fruit or vegetable juices. Some beverages must not be taken into consideration: coffee, tea, milk, soda, wine, and beer. They are too concentrated in hydrophilic substances (which absorb water) to have a hydrating effect.

After several days your average daily intake should be quite clear. If it is below 2.5 liters, you must increase your consumption by drinking enough water to reach 2.5 liters. People who are already drinking 2.5 liters a day should of course continue drinking this much or even increase it slightly.

What to Drink?

The drink designed by nature for human beings is water. We should drink tap water if it is good quality, otherwise bottled mineral water or springwater. It can be sparkling or not, depending on your personal taste. The water you drink may be hot or cold, based on individual preference and vitality. Also recommended are herbal teas such as mint or verbena (with no sweetener added), fruit juice (unsweetened), and vegetable juice.

Make a Plan

Many people forget to drink because they are too involved in their activities. To remedy this it is a good idea to either set up a schedule for drinking regularly at fixed times of the day or fill bottles with the amount of water you need to consume and make it your goal to drink them all by the day's end. By placing them somewhere easily visible, you will be constantly reminded that you need to drink.

One of the first effects of better hydration is a resurgence of energy. But more than that, the lymphatic system will work better; lymph will be abundant and circulate well. It can easily transport toxins and by doing this reinforce the defensive and detoxifying capabilities of the lymph nodes.

🎓 What We've Learned

Lymph has to be continually renewed because it is continually spilling into the bloodstream. When you drink enough you ensure that your body is well hydrated. In this way it will have all the liquid it needs to produce sufficient lymph and ensure proper circulation.

11

Using Medicinal Plants

The oldest evidence for the use of therapeutic medicinal plants by human beings dates back to the fourth millennium BCE. Although it has been enriched over the course of centuries, current knowledge is in large part based on the knowledge of our ancient ancestors.

However, it was not until the seventeenth century CE that the existence of the lymphatic system and its paramount role in the functioning of the body was discovered, so ancient texts from before this time make no mention of plants that have an effect on the lymphatic system. The discovery of such plants is primarily the result of modern research.

In a way that is quite logical, the plants that have a tonic and stimulating effect on the lymphatic vessels are also most often plants that have an effect on the veins. This is because the lymphatic vessels and the veins have many common characteristics. Both ensure return circulation, have contractile walls and valves to encourage circulation, and lack a heart (pump) that propels the fluids they transport. Furthermore, some of the disorders that result from their poor functioning are the same: swelling and feelings of heaviness and fatigue in the legs. In addition, vein and lymphatic circulation are very interdependent and mutually influence each other.

The medicinal plants that act on the lymph vessels and capillaries encourage circulation of lymph. They also stimulate the activity of the lymph nodes, which strengthens the immune system's defenses and helps detoxify the body.

The six medicinal plants I introduce here are divided into two groups. They are taken in either capsule or essential oil form. In addition to their beneficial properties for the lymphatic system, their other properties will also be listed. Each group will allow the selection of plants best suited to individual needs.

PLANTS IN CAPSULES

Capsules are a simple and practical way to take medicinal plants—all you need to do is swallow them with water. When they reach the warm, moist environment of the digestive tract, their walls dissolve and release the active substances of the plant. Recommended dosages are based on a 100 to 500 mg capsule. If in doubt, follow the manufacturer's instructions.

❧ Red Vine (*Vitis vinifera*)

The leaves of red vine have long been used for their tonic effect on the veins and are now also used for their decongestant effect on the lymphatic vessels.

Dosage: 2 capsules, morning and evening, with a large glass of water.

❧ Butcher's Broom (*Ruscus aculeatus*)

An evergreen shrub that is also called box holly, butcher's broom has creeping roots that are used for their vasoconstrictor properties on the veins and lymphatic vessels. They are also anti-inflammatory (therefore a decongestant) and are helpful in the treatment of edemas of the legs.

Dosage: 2 capsules, morning and evening, with a large glass of water.

❧ Yellow Sweet Clover (*Melilotus officinalis*)

This is a small plant known as yellow melilot that has clusters of yellow flowers and grows in fields and on roadsides. The extremely aromatic flowers are used as a tonic for the veins and lymphatic vessels, as a diuretic, and as an antispasmodic for the digestive tract.

Dosage: 2 capsules, morning and evening, with a large glass of water.

PLANTS IN THE FORM OF ESSENTIAL OILS

Essential oils are the oily extracts of plants obtained through distillation, making them very high in active substances. There are several different ways to use them: orally, transdermally, or by inhaling. Essential oils have a very pronounced aroma and taste, so strong that they can be difficult to tolerate over a long period. Because treatment of the lymphatic system with plants is a long-term process, applying them to the skin is a much easier way to proceed.

☝ Good to Know

Essential oils have the virtue of quickly penetrating the skin surface to reach the underlying tissues. Therefore, they easily reach the organ located beneath the place where they have been applied; in this case, the lymph nodes and vessels needing treatment.

Liniment

A liniment is a liquid preparation applied to the skin. Several drops of an essential oil are placed on the skin's surface, then spread by rubbing lightly so it can penetrate.

⚠ Take Note!

Essential oils can be a little aggressive for the skin, so it is preferable to dilute them in oil at a ratio of 10 drops in a tablespoon of oil, or 2 to 3 drops in a teaspoon.

The choice of carrier oils that can be used as a support medium is quite large: apricot kernel, coconut, jojoba, macadamia nut, hazelnut, and sunflower oils are all appropriate individually or in combination.

Macadamia nut oil offers the advantages of stimulating circulation, easily penetrating the skin, and not leaving a greasy sensation. It is preferable to use better-quality oils—in other words, first cold-pressed virgin oils—whenever possible. Make sure you spread the blend over the entire surface you want to treat. One or two applications a day should be enough.

Places to Apply Essential Oils

The application site is chosen based on what you wish to accomplish with this treatment.

A direct effect can be obtained by placing the liniment directly over the exact place you want to treat—for example, over a swollen lymph node, over a ganglial network, or on the legs in the event of a lymphedema in the lower limbs.

Dose

Ten drops of essential oil are necessary for applying as an ointment to the legs, 2 to 3 drops for smaller areas.

An indirect effect that seeks to target the entire lymphatic system can be obtained by letting essential oils penetrate into the areas that have a high number of blood vessels and where the skin surface is thin, which facilitates the entrance of the active principles into the bloodstream. These oils are then brought by the bloodstream into the rest of the body and make contact with the entire lymphatic system. Two zones that respond to these criteria are the elbow crease and the inner surface of the wrist.

The liniment that will be introduced uses both these zones to their best advantage. It has been named an "aromatic perfusion" by its creator, Daniel Pénoël, a French aromatherapist.

The Aromatic Perfusion

Dosage

Place 3 to 5 drops of essential oil in a support substance blend (carrier oil) on the crease of the left elbow. With the inner surface of the right wrist, do four or five rotations over the surface covered with the essential oil to ensure it fully penetrates. Then do the same on the right elbow crease with the left wrist.

Thanks to these movements, the active principles penetrate these two highly receptive areas and then make their way into the lymphatic system.

Following are a few suggestions for plants to use.

❧ Atlas Cedarwood (*Cedrus atlantica*)

The essential oil of this tree from the conifer family has tonic effects on the lymphatic system; it also encourages the healing of wounds. *This plant is contraindicated for pregnant women and children.*

Localized application: 2 to 10 drops blended with carrier oil, one or two applications a day.

Aromatic perfusion: 3 to 4 drops blended with carrier oil on both elbow creases, one or two applications a day.

❧ Cypress (*Cupressus sempervirens*)

Cypress is an easily recognized conifer for its columnar bearing. Cypress essential oil is made from its leafy branches and not with the fruit. Its properties include decongestion of the vein and lymph networks, nerve tonic with rebalancing properties, antispasmodic virtues (cough alleviating) for the respiratory tract.

Localized application: 2 to 10 drops blended with carrier oil, one or two applications a day.

Aromatic perfusion: 3 to 4 drops blended with oil on both elbow creases, one or two applications a day.

❧ Scotch Pine (*Pinus sylvestris*)

Scotch pine grows in colder regions. Its essential oil is made from its needles. Scotch pine is a good lymphatic decongestant and a powerful antiseptic for the respiratory and urinary tracts. It powerfully stimulates the adrenal glands with a cortisone-like effect (anti-inflammatory). Its stimulating effect is sometimes too overwhelming for sensitive individuals to tolerate.

Localized application: 2 to 10 drops blended with carrier oil, one or two applications a day.

Aromatic perfusion: 3 to 4 drops blended with oil on both elbow creases, one or two applications a day.

The beneficial effect of medicinal plants has an effect on not only lymph circulation but also on the lymphatic system's defensive capacities and detoxifying effects.

🎓 What We've Learned

Medicinal plants that are effective on the lymphatic system have an effect that will:

- Tonify the lymphatic vessels
- Stimulate lymph circulation
- Decongest the lymph nodes

12

Restrictive Diets for Rapid Detoxification

While simply changing your diet (see chapter 7) reduces the toxin content of the terrain in general and the lymphatic system in particular, this reduction takes place only gradually. It can take several weeks, if not several months. This expanse of time is too long for someone actually suffering from a disease and who needs to quickly reduce toxin content. To shorten the time it takes for the terrain to be detoxified, a strict, restrictive diet is recommended for a short term; for example a fast, mono diet (monotrophic diet in which only one type of food is eaten), or a vegetable diet.

Why do restrictive diets encourage the elimination of toxins?

During this kind of diet the body receives much less food than usual. However, to function it needs carbohydrates to burn in the muscles, amino acids to repair its tissues, minerals to encourage enzymatic activity, and so on.

Because it is not receiving as much fuel from food, the body is compelled to find this fuel inside itself. During the diet the body will therefore draw the nutrients it needs from its own tissues thanks to a phenomenon called autolysis.

AUTOLYSIS

Autolysis is digestion (*lysis*) of oneself (*auto*) that takes place inside the body. This is a natural phenomenon that can be seen, for example, in tadpoles, which autolyse their own tails to continue their growth into frogs. In the plant kingdom, autolysis by onions of their flowers provides substances that are helpful to the plant's development. It is also due to autolysis that the uterus recovers its normal size after giving birth.

Autolysis takes place thanks to enzymes that act on the various substances that make up our bodies: proteins, fats, carbohydrates, and so on. Fortunately autolysis does not act blindly by attacking all the tissues impartially. If this were the case, all our organs would be damaged in very short order.

To the contrary, the body directs autolysis with intelligence, breaking down the tissues in reverse order of their importance. In other words, the tissues and substances that are the least useful and the least essential to the body in general are subjected to autolysis first, whereas the most important tissues are digested last. First to be attacked are the wastes, then pathological tissues, tumors, and excess fat deposits. It is only after those have been consumed that autolysis goes to work in the more useful tissues of the muscles, skin, and so on.

? Did You Know?

It seems that the vital organs are completely spared by autolysis. This is why, when a person dies of starvation, the autopsy reveals no loss of weight in the "noble organs," such as the brain or heart.

The intelligent breakdown of tissues explains the effectiveness of these strict diets: The enzymes attack all the wastes wherever they find them, breaking them down into usable energies. Toxins are burned to provide energy and broken down into smaller particles that are easier to eliminate. The result is that these wastes disappear from the organic tissues and the terrain gets a deep cleaning. Obviously the quantity of waste the body can eliminate in this way will depend on the length of the diet and the congested state of the terrain.

THE ELIMINATION UPDATE

In conjunction with autolysis there is an elimination update. Because of our eating habits, the quantity of wastes we can eliminate in daily life is less than what we produce. During the restrictive diet the opposite occurs. We are creating less waste than we are eliminating. The body finally has the possibility of getting rid of all the wastes it had been forced to store in the depths of the tissues.

It will make up for this backlog by eliminating all the deep toxins that are broken down by autolysis. These toxins are brought to the surface thanks to blood and lymph and then sent toward the excretory organs. It is, moreover, this rise of toxins that makes the first few days of the diet a little uncomfortable, because they cause blood and lymph to become thicker, thus altering their composition.

Once the wastes have left the tissues and gone back into the blood and lymph, they are transported out of the body by means of the kidneys, liver, or other excretory organs.

⊕ Tips and Tricks

For the elimination update to take place properly, the body's exits must be unobstructed so that the wastes can be expelled. It this is not the case, all you are doing is changing the location of the toxins.

REGENERATION OF THE TISSUE

In addition to autolysis and the elimination update, there is a third phenomenon that takes place during restrictive diets: tissue regeneration.

This tissue regeneration is possible thanks to the elimination update. Because the body no longer has to use the bulk of its energy fighting against the more or less indigestible mass of foods that we ingest continually, it can concentrate on the restoration of the tissues.

Through autolysis substances are removed from tissues of lesser value for the purpose of repairing those tissues that need it. It has often been observed during a diet of this nature that small lesions will repair themselves or start improving, and persistent wounds finally heal. Another explanation for this organic regeneration is the rest that the body is given during the diet.

This is how, thanks to the diet, the ailing lymphatic system can cleanse and recover its strength. The reduction of toxins makes the lymph more fluid and allows it to circulate more easily. The walls of the lymphatic capillaries and vessels get rid of the toxins that were deposited on them, thereby increasing the space in which the lymph can circulate. The muscle fibers distributed in the walls of the lymphatic vessels regenerate and recover their tone. The contractions and dilations of the vessels are restored, and lymphatic circulation recovers its normal speed. The nodes cease to be congested—in other words, clogged by the toxins—which restores their working capabilities. The ancillary lymphatic organs (spleen, thymus, Peyer's patches) are also cleansed and begin to regenerate.

THE RESTRICTIVE DIET IN PRACTICE

The stricter a restrictive diet is, the more effective it will be. Fasts and mono diets are therefore the most detoxifying. In the first case the restriction is total (no food is consumed) and in the second, only a single food is permitted (for example, grapes, carrots, and so on). The diet I'm proposing here, the vegetable cure, is less restrictive than the diets mentioned above but is still quite effective. The restriction of foods is less significant, and the variety of foods you can eat is greater, so more people will be able to stick with it.

The vegetable cure consists of eliminating all foods from your diet except for vegetables. It is similar to a mono diet, but you are eating not one single food but instead one category of food: vegetables.

Meal Composition

Every meal consists solely of vegetables (including fruits that are considered vegetables, such as tomatoes and zucchini), which can be prepared as you choose, in the form of:

- Simple or mixed green salad (thus only a single salad green or with other raw vegetables such as tomatoes, peppers, radishes, and so on)

- Crudités: raw carrots, celery, beets, cabbage, and so on
- Soup: made from one or several vegetables
- Vegetable juice: a single vegetable or several blended

Condiments

The only condiments permitted are a minimal quantity of first cold-pressed virgin oil and sea salt. They can be used together or individually.

Quantity

There is no need to limit the quantity that you eat.

Elimination Aid

To ensure the toxins leave the body, it is a good idea to stimulate the excretory organs (this was covered in chapter 8).

Duration

It is preferable to start with just one day of the cure. Once you have grown accustomed to the process, you can increase it by two or three days, or even more.

Warning Signals

The principal signs that the diet is not being well tolerated and should be interrupted include:

- A great lack of energy and loss of joy
- Too sudden loss of weight
- Breath that smells like acetone (or nail polish remover)

A Summary for Every Day of the Diet

- Eat only vegetables and at all meals, in unlimited amounts.

- Drink as much water and herbal tea (no sweetener) as you like.
- Stimulate the excretory organs with the help of plants.
- Stay active to encourage cellular exchanges and eliminations.

🎓 What We've Learned

Highly restrictive diets, such as mono diets and fasting, trigger autolysis, which digests the toxins present in the tissues. The results of this for the lymphatic system are:

- Purification of the lymph
- Cleansing of the lymphatic vessel walls
- Decongestion of the lymph nodes

13

The Dry Cure

The dry cure is a therapy that aims to accelerate the circulation of lymph by temporarily increasing the "thirst" of the body. The effectiveness of the dry cure can be explained by the close interdependency between lymph and blood and the need to maintain a consistent blood volume.

The body functions properly only when a sufficient amount of blood is circulating through the blood vessels. This volume is based on individual corpulence. It corresponds to a fourteenth of the body's weight, thus around five liters of blood for someone who weighs 70 kilos (about 150 pounds).

The body actively works to maintain this constant volume, which can vary over time. It increases when we drink a lot and is then corrected by the kidneys, which eliminate excess liquid in the form of urine. We urinate more when we consume more liquid.

When, to the contrary, we don't drink enough, blood volume diminishes. Drinking too little means drinking less than the 2.5 liters a day that we lose in urine (1.5 liters), sweat (0.5 liter), exhaled air (0.4 liter), and stool (0.1 liter). These 2.5 liters must be restored to our body to keep blood volume normal.

To ensure that the quantity of liquid it needs is given to it, the body triggers feelings of thirst as soon as blood volume starts to shrink. Some people are not aware of feeling thirsty and drink very little. Over the long term, their blood volume can become dangerously reduced. The body has to seek another way to restore its blood volume, and it finds it in the lymphatic system. From this lymph the blood circulatory system can draw the fluid it needs.

To maintain blood volume, lymph naturally spills into it every day by way of the subclavian veins. But in an emergency, which is the case when there is an insufficient amount of blood in the vessels, this spilling of lymph becomes more profuse. The output can double or triple, which means that a lot more lymph than usual will be poured into the bloodstream, thereby permitting the reestablishment of the proper blood volume.

This increased output benefits not only the bloodstream but also lymphatic circulation, which accelerates with all the advantages that this entails.

By accelerating, lymph sweeps out and carries away toxins that have been stagnating on the walls of the lymphatic vessels, in the same way that a stream whose flow increases carries off waste that has been stagnating on its banks. The lymph pours the toxins it carries more quickly into the bloodstream, which carries it to the excretory organs to be discarded out of the body.

In the lymph nodes the increased flow of lymph increases the number of toxins and microbes they can intercept, which they consequently neutralize and destroy. The result is a more intense purification of the lymph. The accelerated passage of lymph through the nodes also rids them of toxins and microbe corpses that may be stagnating there. They can therefore regenerate from this and become more effective in actively defending the body.

This intensification of the outflow of lymph into the bloodstream requires a higher amount of the interstitial fluid removed by the lymphatic capillaries, but this is also a good thing. The removed interstitial fluid goes into the lymphatic system with the wastes taken from the organic tissues it bathes, resulting in a more extensive detoxification of the deep tissues. Furthermore, this increased removal of interstitial fluid contributes to reducing the swelling of tissues so that any edemas formed due to slowed lymphatic circulation can be reabsorbed.

THE PRACTICE OF THE CURE

The reduction of blood volume can be obtained only by a strong limitation of fluid intake. Two forms of this cure are possible.

The Dry Fast

During a normal fast, all foods are completely removed, but water and herbal teas are permissible. In a dry fast, one doesn't eat or drink. This is a much more stringent restriction that obviously cannot be maintained for very long.

The Dry Diet

The dry diet is one during which you don't drink anything. It is not a fast, however, as foods can be eaten. The foods chosen have very low water content:

- Nuts: walnuts (3.3 percent water), almonds (4.7 percent water), hazelnuts (4.8 percent water), Brazil nuts (5.3 percent water)
- Various crackers: wheat crackers (8.5 percent water), crispbread crackers (9 percent water)
- Dried fruits: dates (20 percent water), raisins (24 percent water), dried apricots (24 percent water)
- Bread (34–37 percent water)

The advantage of the dry diet is that eating is permitted, which is reassuring for some people. However, the foods in question are dry and can rapidly make you thirsty, which will exacerbate what you are already feeling due to depriving yourself of liquids.

Length of the Cures

In the beginning either the dry fast or the dry diet should last no more than twenty-four hours. A break of seven to ten days is then necessary to allow the body to recover before repeating the cure. In fact, even a one-day cure has a beneficial effect on the lymphatic system, but this benefit is only partial. To get a more complete and deeper effect, you must repeat the cure several times.

The repetitions allow you to get familiar with the cure and learn how to better understand your body's reactions to the restricted intake of liquid. If you are able to tolerate these cures well, their duration can be increased to a maximum of two days for the dry fast and three days for the dry diet. An intermediary break of a week to ten days is necessary between each cure.

⚠ Take Note!

For the sake of safety, oversight of fasts by a naturopath or fasting specialist is recommended, particularly in the beginning. Listen to your body and never force yourself to fast to the detriment of your health, physical or mental.

Warning Signals

The principal signs that a fast or diet is not being tolerated by your body and that you must end it are:

- Severe loss of energy
- Drop in blood pressure
- Feeling of mental or physical malaise
- Rapid weight loss
- Breath smells like acetone

Starting the Cure

Dry cures are more effective if the body is prepared for the strong restrictions awaiting it. By definition, intake is completely absent in the dry fast and extremely reduced in the dry diet, so the person on the cure will eat very little.

Preparing for the cure doesn't have to be dry. There should, however, be a significant reduction in intake of food and water, which is easily done by eliminating heavy foods (meat, fish, dairy, eggs, grains, pasta) and eating only light foods, thus fruits and vegetables.

The day before the cure, normal meals should be eaten but consist of only plant-based foods. The vegetables can be consumed raw, cooked, in juice, or in soup. Oil for salad dressing and salt are permitted. The fruits, similarly, are to be eaten raw, juiced, or cooked (but with no sugar added).

Even if large quantities of fruits and vegetables are eaten on this day, these are very light foods that will prepare the body to receive even less.

Ending the Cure

It is also a good idea to follow the fruit and vegetable diet on the day after the dry cure. The goal is to prevent overworking the body by giving it heavy foods directly following the cure. It needs a transitional period to acclimate to the resumption of a normal diet.

Ending the dry cure also means starting to drink again. On the first day following, it is recommended not only to drink but to drink a lot. This is because the body will need a lot of liquid, as it has been totally deprived during the day or days of the cure, and it is the way normal blood volume is reestablished quickly, albeit higher than normal. This increases the blood pressure and thus the force with which blood enters the excretory organs. This greatly facilitates the elimination of toxins that the cure has extracted from the depths of the body.

SUPPLEMENTS TO THE CURE

Abstention of water is the central aspect of the cure, but there are other elements that greatly enhance the process.

Physical Exercise

During the cure the larger spillage of lymph into the bloodstream increases toxins in the blood and thickens it, causing blood circulation to slow, which reduces metabolic rates and thereby the detoxifying effect of the cure. To counteract this, it is important to perform sufficient physical activity during both the dry diet and the dry fast. Thanks to muscle contraction, the speed of the bloodstream will be maintained and even slightly accelerated, which will ensure good filtering of toxins by the excretory organs. In the final analysis, the blood and lymph remain cleaner, the body is well oxygenated, and the person taking the cure feels much lighter and fitter.

Physical activities should be practiced gently but with enough intensity to cause a slight feeling of breathlessness. This will force the heart to beat harder and more quickly, which increases the speed of circulation.

Some recommended physical activities include:

- Walking, partially uphill
- Long bike rides
- Tennis
- Dancing

Medicinal Plants

The dry cure will create a much larger transport of toxins into the excretory organs. It is therefore imperative that these organs are capable of handling a massive arrival of toxins. They have to be able to filter them out of the blood and eliminate them so that they actually leave the body. Otherwise the toxins that have left the depths of the tissues will end up near the surface in the bloodstream. The body will not be rid of them. It is therefore essential to ensure that the excretory organs are fully functioning.

Two excretory organs play a particularly important role in dry cures: the liver and the intestines. These are the specific organs that handle colloidal wastes, the exact toxins that lymph transports. Some medicinal plants, including alder buckthorn, mallow, and dandelion, act on both organs at the same time.

Because this is a dry cure, the plant chosen should be swallowed with the least amount of water possible. This means plant infusions cannot be recommended, but capsules or mother tinctures can. In both forms a small amount of water will certainly be needed, but it can be minimal.

To make certain the liver and intestines are wide open for the cure, it is recommended to take the plant you select the entire week before the cure, then continue taking it during the cure, and then another three days after the cure is complete.

Here are two sample options:

- Alder buckthorn in a mother tincture: 20 to 30 drops three times a day, with a minimum of water
- Mallow in capsules: 1 or 2 capsules* three times a day with a minimum of water

Dosage should allow one or two stools a day.

Cure Plan

Days 1–5	
Normal diet	Medicinal plant for the liver/intestines
Day 6	
Fruit-vegetable diet	Medicinal plant for the liver/intestines

---

*Recommended dosage is based on a 100 to 500 mg capsule. If in doubt, follow the manufacturer's instructions.

Day 7	
Dry fast or dry diet	Medicinal plant for the liver/intestines
Day 8	
Fruit-vegetable diet, copious fluids	Medicinal plant for the liver/intestines
Days 9–11	
Normal diet	Medicinal plant for the liver/intestines

THE WATER CURE AND THE DRY CURES ARE NOT IN CONFLICT

Isn't it contradictory to recommend a dry cure in this chapter and a hydration cure in chapter 10 as two methods for supporting the lymphatic system? How can two opposing methods have the same effect?

These two methods are opposed only in appearance. Both have a beneficial effect on lymph circulation, but with a different angle of attack. The water cure acts on the entrance of lymph into the lymphatic network, the dry cure on its exit from this same network.

An *increase* in the volume of water ingested increases blood pressure and thus increases the pressure pushing the interstitial fluid into the lymphatic capillaries. When this pressure is high there is an acceleration in the circulation of lymph.

A *reduction* of water consumed lowers the overall volume of blood and thereby increases the necessity for the lymphatic system to surrender lymph to reestablish proper blood volume. Greater quantities of lymph will enter the bloodstream at the subclavian veins, which has the effect of accelerating the speed of lymph circulation.

🎓 What We've Learned

The dry cure consists of drinking virtually nothing during a short period. The dehydration that results reduces blood volume, which forces the lymphatic system to draw interstitial fluid to travel back up through it in the form of lymph until it reaches the bloodstream. The result of this is a beneficial acceleration of lymph circulation, which decongests the lymphatic vessels and lymph nodes.

14

Lymphatic Drainage Massage

Lymphatic draining is a massage technique perfected during the 1930s by Emil and Estrid Vodder. Observing that people suffering from chronic colds had swollen lymph nodes, the couple suspected the nodes might be a means of healing these patients. Because standard massage had no effect, they explored another way to proceed. Using an intuitive approach and following the sensations of their hands, they discovered that slow, gentle movements contrary to those of traditional massage were effective. Over time they perfected their massage technique, and because it worked specifically on the lymphatic system and encouraged the flow of lymph, it was called "lymphatic draining."

EFFECT OF LYMPHATIC DRAINING

Lymphatic draining makes it possible to remove congestion from swollen lymph nodes. It encourages the circulation of lymph and can even accelerate it. It also encourages the entry of interstitial fluid into the lymphatic capillaries and thereby reduces stagnation caused by the accumulation of fluid in the interstitial space (edema).

This technique is therefore most helpful for people suffering from diseases of the lymphatic system. It requires precise knowledge of the location of the lymph nodes and the course of the lymphatic vessels, as it is over them that the massage takes place. Practice of this massage requires extensive study to do it correctly. It is therefore recommended to consult therapists trained in this modality.

✚ Tips and Tricks

It is possible to perform lymphatic self-massage, but this is something you would have to learn. The advantage of this approach is that the person involved can self-drain as a complete treatment or alternate with sessions provided by a professional.

How is lymphatic draining different from standard massage?

DISTINCTIVE FEATURES OF STANDARD MASSAGE

Western massage consists of working deeply on the muscle mass and organs to accelerate their blood circulation. Various manipulations used for this purpose include kneading (wringing, rolling, treading with the feet), pressure (crushing, pounding), percussion (with the fingers, sides of the hands, fists), friction, and vibration.

These different massage manipulations are done forcefully to ensure their effects go deep and are performed at a rather rapid speed and rhythm. They are characterized by their intensity.

THE DISTINCTIVE FEATURES OF LYMPHATIC DRAINING

Lymphatic draining is a slow massage, corresponding to the slowness that is characteristic of lymphatic circulation. It is also very gentle because the lymphatic capillaries are quite thin and delicate.

The light touch with which the movements are performed are based on the fact that lymphatic draining works almost entirely on the skin's surface. It causes this surface to slide back and forth over the underlying tissues from left to right and diagonally. The purpose of these manipulations is to stretch the filaments connecting the portals of the lymphatic capillaries to the neighboring tissues (skin). When they receive the signal to open this way, these portals expand, allowing interstitial fluid to enter the capillaries more easily.

The effect on the surface also stimulates the lymphatic capillaries and vessels as well as lymph circulation. The manipulations are adapted to mimic the characteristics of the lymphatic system—light pressure, specific intensity (not too weak or strong), and at a predetermined speed corresponding with the vasodilation and vasoconstriction of the lymphatic vessels. The movements are applied repeatedly to small surface areas before moving on to the next area. This process is continued along the entire length of the trajectory being treated. Depending on the case, these manipulations may be circular movements—over a node, for example—or pumping movements to draw the lymph out of congested areas.

Lymphatic draining distinguishes itself from standard massage because it concentrates its efforts on the surface and not on the depths of the body. The surface areas involved are circumscribed and not extensive. The gentle nature of lymphatic draining does not accelerate the speed of blood circulation, which is a precise intention in standard massage.

INDICATIONS FOR LYMPHATIC DRAINING

The health disorders for which lymphatic draining is recommended are those connected with the three major functions of the lymphatic system.

Circulatory Function

Lymphedema, water retention, heavy legs, swollen ankles, cramps, poor venous circulation, acute sprains, excess weight, cellulitis, headaches, migraines, scarring.

Immune System, Anti-Infection, and Anti-Inflammation

Overall immune system weakness: infections, colds, otitis, sinusitis, angina, conjunctivitis, acne, wounds, varicose ulcers; and painful inflammations such as rheumatism, osteoarthritis, tendinitis, neuritis, myalgia, inflamed nodes, and so on.

Detoxifying Function

Because the overload of toxins is the source of most disease, lymphatic draining takes effect on all the disorders mentioned above as well as on cardiovascular disease, respiratory illness, skin disorders, fatigue, anxiety, vulnerability to stress, depressive tendencies, and more.

LYMPHATIC DRAINING IN PRACTICE

Generally speaking, treatment begins with one or two sessions a week, no more. This is because the relaunch of lymphatic circulation continues to manifest for some time after the session, and sessions taking place too close to one another will set a lot of toxins into motion, which can have unpleasant effects (feelings of malaise, headaches, and so on). The sessions can then continue at a slower frequency determined by the practitioner and based on the patient and the evolution of the disorder—for example, one session a week, then one every two weeks, and so forth.

🎓 What We've Learned

Lymphatic draining is a special massage method applied to lymphatic vessels and lymph nodes. These slow, gentle manipulations encourage:

- Entrance of interstitial fluid into the lymphatic vessels
- Peristaltic movement of the lymphatic vessels
- Decongestion of the nodes

15

Foot Reflexology

Foot reflexology, like all lymphatic draining methods, is a therapeutic approach that makes it possible to work directly on the lymphatic system. It can also reach lymphatic organs in the depths of the body, such as the Pecquet cistern, tonsils, and spleen. Foot reflexology acts at a distance on the organs, via the intermediary of the nerves, by massaging the reflex zones that are located primarily on the soles of the feet.

There are, however, a few points on the top of the feet and on the ankles; this is the case for the reflex zones connected to the lymphatic system.

Foot reflexology zones are small areas on the skin's surface that are terminal points for nerves from different organs. Each organ is therefore connected to a specific zone of the skin. Because of this linkage, the deterioration of the health of an organ will have repercussions on the reflex zone; it will become sensitive and even painful to the touch. The degree of pain the reflex zone experiences is proportionate to the seriousness of the disorders suffered by the organ.

However, the connection between reflex zone and organ is not unidirectional. The massage of a reflex zone also sends information to the organ connected to it. This is indeed a reflex action; the organ reacts automatically to the stimulation transmitted by the nerve. The effect of this stimulation is to activate the blood circulation of the organ involved, stimulating elimination of the toxins that are congesting it and preventing the organ from functioning properly. Reflex massage, therefore, intensifies the work of the lymphatic organs whose reflex zones are massaged. This improves not only lymph circulation but the defensive and detoxifying capacities of the lymphatic system as well.

MASSAGING THE REFLEX ZONES OF THE LYMPHATIC SYSTEM

Massage of the foot reflex zones is done with the help of the thumb or phalanx joint of a finger, generally the index finger. The reflex zone selected is then rubbed in a circular motion with varying pressure. Smearing the zone with lotion beforehand will make the massage easier. In the beginning the treatment should last only a few minutes (two to five). It should be performed on both feet given the fact that all organs have two reflex zones, one on each foot.

The location of the lymphatic system reflex zones is shown in the illustrations that follow in this chapter. A small anatomical explanation is also provided. The sense of touch will allow you to complete this information and find exactly where the reflex zone is located. The zones that need to be massaged are generally painful when pressure is applied to them.

The pain caused by toxins that have collected in the reflex zones can make the zone hurt even when it is not being massaged, indicating that toxins have accumulated in not only the ailing organ but in its reflex zones as well.

In the beginning, massage of the reflex zones is performed gently so as not to cause the patient too much pain or release too many toxins at one time. When a lot of toxins enter the blood at the same time, the body can be temporarily overwhelmed and manifest a variety of disorders, such as headache, nausea, irritability, insomnia, or fever. These disorders are not very serious, but they are unpleasant, so it is better to avoid them. Therefore, this circular rubbing massage technique should be applied more strongly only gradually so as to increase the strength of the massage without reaching the discomfort zone.

The duration of reflex zone massage increases over time. From two to three minutes per zone in the beginning to ten minutes, then to twenty or thirty minutes. One massage session a day is the normal rhythm, but two or three shorter sessions a day have also proved beneficial. The stimulating effect of a session, which necessarily fades over time, is thereby relaunched the same day with more sessions.

The first effects on the lymphatic system can appear quite quickly, after a week or two. Several months are needed, though, to get profound results.

Reflex zone massage is something everyone can perform, and the technique is easy to learn and self-administer. It is also possible to turn to one of the many therapists who practice this treatment.

OUTLINE

- Reflex zone of the spleen. This area stimulates this organ's functioning. The zone is located on the bottom of only the left foot.

Left foot

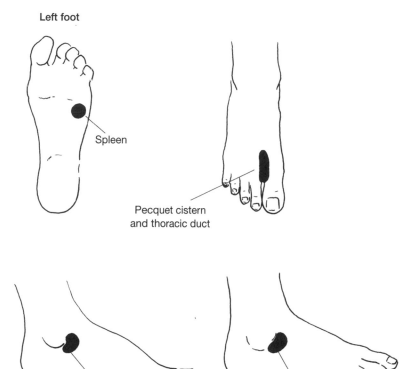

Spleen

Pecquet cistern
and thoracic duct

Lymph nodes of
the abdomen

Lymph nodes, upper
half of the body

Reflex zones of the lymphatic system

- Reflex zone of the Pecquet cistern and the thoracic duct. This area stimulates the circulation of lymph in these two organs and thereby in the rest of the body. It is located on both feet, in the hollow spot between the first and second metatarsal bones.
- Reflex zone of the abdominal lymph nodes. This area drains the legs, abdomen, and pelvis. It is located on the

top of both feet in a small hollow just before the inside of the anklebone.

- Reflex zone of the thorax lymph nodes. This area drains the upper half or the abdomen and the head. It is on top of both feet in the small hollow just before the outside of the anklebone.

🎓 What We've Learned

Several reflex zones on the feet are connected to the lymphatic system. By massaging these zones regularly we can directly sustain and intensify lymphatic action.

16

Deep and Whole-Body Breathing

The right and left thoracic ducts, the largest lymphatic vessels, collect lymph coming from all over the body and transport it into the subclavian veins so that it can reach the blood circulatory system. This means that smooth functioning of the thoracic ducts is essential. Any stagnation in them will slow lymph circulation throughout the lymphatic network.

The thoracic ducts are located between the lungs, two organs that can significantly support and sustain lymph circulation in this area of the body. In fact, the presence of the thoracic ducts between both lungs makes them sensitive to the opening and closing movements of the thoracic cage.

When we inhale, the lungs increase in size and compress the thoracic ducts, thereby pushing forward the lymph they contain. When we exhale, the lungs deflate, giving the thoracic ducts more space, which allows them to dilate. Consequently, they suck up lymph located lower down in the network, which has the result of making it circulate.

The lungs therefore encourage lymphatic circulation by applying pressure to the thoracic ducts, but this happens only when we take deep breaths. As a rule we do not breathe deeply

most of the time—in fact, our breath is often quite shallow—
with the result that the dilations and contractions of the lungs
are weak.

The size of the airstream we inhale when we are quietly
sitting at a desk, for example, is not elevated. It is in the neigh-
borhood of half a liter and does not cause any visible change
in the size of the lungs. But it is entirely possible for us to
breathe in more air as we would if we were involved in some
kind of physical activity. This additional air could be any-
where between one to three liters, so it clearly changes the size
of the lungs.

While the lungs can dilate much more strongly than usual
on an inhale, they also reduce again on an exhale. When we
finish breathing out with the exhalation of about half a liter of
air, it is still possible for us to exhale more air (the air reserves)
contained in the lower depths of the lungs. The volume of this
air is about one to two liters.

Lung capacity thus totals approximately five to six liters.
This is an elevated volume of air. By entering and leaving the
lungs it creates significant movements of compression and
release in the thoracic ducts, creating the beneficial effects of
breathing on lymphatic circulation.

There are two different ways of breathing based on the
extent of the respiratory movements: deep breathing and
whole-body breathing.

BREATHING IN PRACTICE

While breathing is often automatic thanks to the autonomic
nervous system, it is possible to use the breath to our greater
advantage.

Deep Breathing

Deep breathing is also called diaphragmatic or belly breathing as it primarily uses the diaphragm. This dome- or umbrella-shaped muscle forms the dividing wall separating the thoracic cavity from the abdominal cavity. Therefore, the upper surface of the diaphragm is in contact with the heart and lungs and its lower surface with the liver, stomach, and spleen.

It's thanks to the diaphragm that we can inhale and exhale deeply when we wish to intensify our respiratory movements. By pushing toward the bottom we open the lungs, and by pushing up, we close them.

Before we examine deep breathing, it would be a good idea to first understand the way we usually breathe, thanks to the following exercise.

@ Exercise 1: Becoming Aware of Your Breathing

Lie on your back on a level surface, with a bolster beneath your knees to elevate them. Then place one hand on your chest and the other on your belly just below the navel and observe yourself breathing. Most commonly only the chest is moving and the belly remains still. This is the way most people breathe over the course of the day. It is called thoracic breathing.

Now, let's look at deep breathing.

@ Exercise 2: Deep Breathing

This is a continuation of exercise 1, with an intentional increase in the scope of your breathing movements. After breathing in through the nose, breathe out through the nose slowly and deeply by pulling in your belly. Your diaphragm will contract and rise inside the abdomen. Once you have stopped exhaling, start inhaling. Breathe in by pushing your belly down and forward. The diaphragm will dilate and descend inside the abdomen.

With this exercise it is easy to see that the volume of air taken in and released is much larger. This is because more air is filling the bottom of the lungs. The hand placed flat over your belly allows you to follow the diaphragm's movements of reduction and expansion.

The complete exercise consists of taking a series of these deep inhalations and exhalations over a period of two to three minutes.

✚ Tips and Tricks

The rhythm of a deep-breathing exercise should be slow so as to give your lungs the time they need to fill and empty completely, but not so slow that you are holding your breath. In short, it should have a rhythm that allows you to feel comfortable for the entire exercise.

Start by doing one session of one to two minutes each day, then move on to two or three daily sessions, and gradually extend to five minutes. With practice the exercise will become easier, and at that point you can move on to whole-body breathing.

Whole-Body Breathing

In deep breathing the goal is to replace exhaled air with that inhaled, but no more. The dilations and contractions of the lungs provide a beneficial influence on the lymphatic circulation, but the extent of the breath can be increased yet further if additional air is introduced during the inhalation. In practice you need to proceed as explained in the next exercise.

⊚ Exercise 3: Whole-Body Breathing

Stretch out lying down as in the previous exercise. After a deep exhale, gently inhale to replace the air you just exhaled. When the lungs are back to where they were at the beginning, don't stop there but continue inhaling by drawing in the maximum amount of air possible to completely fill the lungs. The lifting of the thorax and slight elevation of the shoulders this causes have the happy consequence of swelling the lungs even more. It is the addition of this extra bit of air that distinguishes whole-body breathing from deep breathing.

The sessions should be done one to three times a day with a series of breaths over a span of two to five minutes, if not longer.

To avoid triggering an adverse reaction by hyperventilating, the breathing rhythm has to be comfortable for the person doing it—neither two slow nor too fast. By staying aware of the way it makes you feel, you will be able to find the rhythm that suits you best.

A prone position is best for learning how to breathe. However, once you have learned how to do it properly, these exercises can be performed while sitting or standing. This allows you to practice them at different times during the day: while sitting in your office or watching TV, waiting in a line, on public transportation, and so forth.

🎓 What We've Learned

The swelling and relaxation of the lungs during exercises of deep or whole-body breathing applies rhythmic pressure on the thoracic duct and the lymphatic vessels of the torso, which accelerates lymph circulation throughout the lymphatic network.

17

Trampoline Exercises

Jumping on a trampoline, also called a rebounder, is a very popular game for children, but this practice has been revealed to provide valuable assistance for accelerating lymph circulation and decongesting the lymphatic system of adults.

WHAT HAPPENS IN A JUMP

The stretched canvas and springs of a trampoline increase the scope of each movement so that with each jump you go higher and then lower. The alternation of these contrary movements influences bodily fluids, particularly lymph.

When you bounce your body rises suddenly and quickly. While this accelerated movement propels your body upward, it exerts an opposite force on the lymph. It is as if it were pushed toward the bottom because it didn't manage to follow the movement of the body. The phenomenon is the same as when a plane takes off. The airplane is moving forward at a high speed, but the passengers clearly feel a force in the opposite direction that flattens them against their seats. We can feel this same sensation on a seesaw or on a swing in an upward arc.

To provide a more visual illustration of what is happening, let's observe what happens to someone with long hair when jumping on a trampoline. As the person goes up, the body rises but the hair does not; rather, it is pushed town and flattened against the head. Similar processes take place physiologically. During the bounce the lymph is pushed downward, which has the effect of immediately closing the lymphatic valves.

But hardly have they closed when the body begins falling back toward the trampoline. This descent is also sudden and quick. It propels the body downward, but the lymph is sent in the opposite direction. It's as if it couldn't manage to follow the body's descent, so it drags behind, which pushes it upward along its path.

The phenomenon is the same when an elevator descends quickly from a high floor. You get the impression of falling into a void and a sensation of stomach-turning. It's as if the heart couldn't manage to follow and stayed where it was. To use the image of the hair again, when someone jumps to the bottom of a wall, long hair doesn't hang down but is instead pushed upward. The direction of this thrust, though, is the same as that of the circulation of lymph in the lymphatic system. Lymph is therefore prompted to advance, which opens the lymphatic valves.

Over the course of a trampoline session, the contrary pressures applied to the lymph connect together and follow every two to three seconds. In this way lymph is pushed back and forth with regard to lymph circulation. However, the backward movement of the lymph is always immediately halted, as the valves close as soon as they feel a backward surge.

Lymph is, therefore, definitively and continuously projected forward toward its eventual exit. Its advance through the lymphatic vessels is encouraged. The segments in the lymphatic system where lymph is stagnating are decongested, and those where circulation was slow will see an acceleration. Its circulation speed will be increased throughout the entire time you are on the trampoline and for some time afterward. Repeating this activity regularly is a good way to gradually restore good lymphatic circulation.

Jumping on the trampoline also has a beneficial effect on valves and muscle fibers responsible for the vasoconstriction and dilation of the lymphatic vessels. They work for the entire duration of the trampoline session. Every two or three seconds the valves open and close and the muscle fibers contract. This intense activity restores their tone, which makes them better able to guarantee proper circulation of the lymph.

☝ Good to Know

The effects gained from using the trampoline are the same as those created by physical exercise. The main difference is that trampoline sessions do not require the muscles to work as hard as they would during exercise and similar physical activities. For this reason they are especially indicated for people who are not capable of performing intense physical activity over any length of time.

TRAMPOLINES IN PRACTICE

Trampolines designed for indoor use are sold in a variety of places. They are lower and generally smaller in circumference than outdoor trampolines, so you can bounce on them without worrying about hitting the ceiling if you are indoors. The outdoor trampolines used by children work perfectly well, especially if they have netting around the perimeter to guard against accidental jumps or falls off the edge.

The descriptions I've given thus far may have given the impression that you must make big jumps, but that is not necessary for good results. Small jumps are also beneficial. They are even better for people with a weaker sense of balance or those who are affected by lymphedemas. This latter group of people can also use compression socks (see chapter 18) to perform these exercises.

Following are two different ways to use the trampoline to stimulate lymphatic circulation.

Simply Lift Your Heels

Stand up straight on the trampoline with your feet slightly apart, knees slightly bent, arms relaxed. Lift up your heels while standing on your tiptoes on the trampoline. The impulse will come from the front ends of your feet, but they will not break contact with the trampoline. As soon as your heels go back down and touch the trampoline, raise them again. Link these movements together in a rhythm that you find pleasant, one you can master without too much effort. In the beginning sessions should last only two to three minutes, but with training they can be extended to five, ten, and even fifteen minutes. Some people may even do thirty-minute sessions.

⚠ Take Note!

It is important to approach trampoline work with good sense; in other words, take it gradually. By rushing things you run the risk of creating the opposite of what you intend. The lymphatic system will become tired and lymph circulation will slow as a result.

Gentle Jumps

The second way to use the trampoline is a little more dynamic. Stand up straight on the trampoline with your feet slightly apart, knees slightly bent, arms relaxed. In this exercise your feet will come entirely off the trampoline. Make small jumps of about four to five inches off the trampoline. Establish a comfortable rhythm and do this for two to three minutes. Once you feel you have mastered this you can increase the time of the sessions to five or ten minutes, then fifteen or longer.

The same rules apply here as in the exercise based on lifting your heels. Use your common sense and don't overdo it. Higher jumps than those described here are possible over time.

🎓 What We've Learned

The alternating upward and downward motion of jumps on the trampoline will push lymph forward in the lymphatic vessels. In addition, the changing pressure will place repeated demands on the valves. This will strengthen them and thereby encourage better lymph circulation.

18

Compression Therapy

Compression therapy is indicated only for individuals suffering from lymphedema, whether the edemas appear in the arms or legs. It adds excellent value to the basic therapies but is not enough on its own to provide satisfying results.

The method consists of applying permanent pressure on the parts of the body that are swollen by lymphedema, to prevent them from swelling more by collecting interstitial fluid. This pressure is applied through the use of clothing known as compression sleeves or stockings—leggings, tights, or socks for the legs, or sleeves for the arms. The clothes are manufactured with a tight elastic fabric. Because they are stretchy, they can be put on the ailing limb, but once in place, they partially go back to their original size, hence their compressive effect. This pressure can be light or strong, depending on the desired results.

Compression garments are sometimes mistakenly called restraining garments. Restraining garments do exist, but they are not elastic. Therefore, the pressure they provide is not constant but appears only in reaction to muscle contractions; for example, they prevent swelling of the legs that can happen while walking by supplying passive resistance.

Compression sleeves and stockings have to be adjusted perfectly. They should not be too loose, or they will have no effect. But they cannot be too tight as that could hinder blood circulation. In addition, overly high pressure on the blood vessels causes an increase in the infusion of serum into the interstitial area. The volume of interstitial fluid will increase—a volume that is already too high as shown by the existence of a lymphedema. Therefore, the choice of compression stockings or sleeves should be guided by professionals, and their dimensions should be regularly verified and adjusted for the lymphedema.

Compression garments are intended to be worn during the day, especially when physical activity, long periods of standing, or air travel are anticipated. These have a tendency to increase fluid volume in the limbs, which are vulnerable to edemas. Compression clothing is also recommended for after lymphatic draining sessions to prolong the effects of treatment.

Treatments using these items are long-term treatments. They help restrict the accumulation of interstitial fluid in the limbs and prevent edemas from becoming chronic.

Compression garments are not worn at night, so as to leave the body free.

🎓 What We've Learned

The use of compression stockings or sleeves:

- Limits fluid collection in the limbs
- Prevents tissues from swelling in the event of lymphedema

Conclusion

Recent studies of the lymphatic system have revealed to an even greater extent the major role it plays in our good health.

The circulation of nutrients, hormones, lymphocytes, and so forth in the body is accomplished not only thanks to the bloodstream but also in large part due to the lymph. The lymphatic system and excretory organs work together to detoxify the body.

A considerable part of the cellular terrain is made up of lymph—vascular lymph and interstitial lymph. The lymphatic system is not a minor player in the immune defenses but instead constitutes the principal part of the immune system.

Although located in the depths of our bodies, the lymphatic system is accessible to therapies used in natural medicine. We have at our disposal simple methods for sustaining and strengthening it, thus keeping the lymphatic system healthy and maintaining overall health.

Glossary

adenoids: Lymphoidal tissue located in the back of the nose.

adenopathy: Swelling of a lymph node.

adipocyte: Cell that specializes in the storage of fat.

agglutination: The process during which two different substances adhere to each other.

alveoli: Pockets at the tips of the bronchioles where gas exchanges take place.

amino acids: Molecules that combine to form proteins. There are nine essential amino acids.

antibodies: Blood proteins produced by a lymphocyte to destroy the microbes possessing the corresponding antigen.

antigen: A toxin or other foreign substance that triggers antibody production by the lymphocytes.

appendix: A small pouch surrounded by lymphatic tissue, located between the small and large intestines.

arteriosclerosis: The hardening and thickening of the artery walls accompanied by plaque created by deposits of fatty waste.

autolysis: The digestion or breakdown (*lysis*) by the body of its own tissues (*auto*) thanks to enzymes.

axillary: Medical term for armpit.

capillary: An extremely thin vessel that irrigates the deep tissue. There are blood capillaries and lymph capillaries.

catarrh: Copious secretions created by inflammation of the mucous membranes.

cecum: Beginning of the ascending colon (large intestine).

chyle: Milky fluid made up of fat and lymph that is created by the transformation of foods in the small intestine.

chyliferous vessels: These transport chyle.

collecting ducts: Large lymphatic vessels that collect the lymph transported there by several smaller lymphatic vessels.

colloid: A mixture of one or two gelatinous substances that are not chemically combined.

creatinine: A waste product created by the breakdown of proteins in muscles during normal wear and tear.

crystalloidal: Substances that have a hard consistency, like a crystal.

drainage: The deliberate intensification of eliminations intended to rid the body of toxins.

embolism: The obstruction of a blood vessel by a blood clot.

enzyme: A substance that activates chemical transformations in the body.

excretory organs: Technically called emunctory organs, these are the organs responsible for filtering toxins out of the bloodstream and expelling them from the body. The five excretory organs are the liver, intestines, kidneys, skin, and lungs.

extracellular fluid: The bodily fluid that surrounds cells. Also called interstitial fluid when it is outside the blood.

germinal centers: Groups of cells inside lymph nodes whose role is to produce lymphocytes.

hemorrhoid: Dilation of the veins in the anus and rectum.

Hodgkin's lymphoma: Cancer that starts in white blood cells (lymphocytes), which then grow out of control.

hydrostatic pressure: Pressure exerted by a fluid at rest on adjacent bodies due to the force of gravity.

inguinal: Related to the groin, the hollow that separates the abdomen from the upper leg.

interstitial fluid: The fluid that fills spaces between the cells and is outside the blood. It is referred to as extracellular serum or fluid.

intracellular: Bodily fluid found inside cells.

lactic acid: Acid that forms in the muscles following sustained effort.

leucocyte: From the Greek word for white (*leuco*); a white blood corpuscle.

leukemia: Cancer of the bone marrow that causes profound changes to blood composition by creating an excess of white blood cells.

lithiasis: The presence of deposits, often mineral-like, in the ducts and vessels.

lymph: Clear fluid that circulates in the lymphatic vessels. It is also called white blood as opposed to the red blood circulating in the blood vessels.

lymphangion: A segment of the lymphatic vessel equipped with two one-directional valves that help propel lymph forward.

lymphocyte: A lymphatic cell that plays a fundamental role in the body's immune system; it is essential for the body's defenses.

lymphedema: Accumulation of lymph in the lymphatic vessels and interstitial compartment, manifested as swelling.

lysis: The decomposition of organic substances with the help of specialized enzymes.

macrophage: A large (macro) cell of the immune system that swallows microbes and destroys them by digesting them.

metastasis: The formation of a cancerous tumor from cancer cells that separated from a tumor located elsewhere in the body.

morbific: Something that causes sickness.

node: A small swelling on the trajectory of a lymphatic vessel consisting of the cells responsible for neutralizing toxins and germs.

non-Hodgkin's lymphoma: A tumor of a lymph node caused by an abnormal increase in the number of B or T lymphocytes.

nutrients: Substances necessary for the building and functioning of the body—proteins, lipids, carbohydrates, omega-3 fatty acids, vitamins, minerals, trace elements, and so forth.

organelle: A small organ located inside a cell.

osmosis: The transfer of fluid from a lesser concentrated milieu—in other words, one that is low in suspended solid particles—toward a more concentrated fluid, until the balance of liquids is equalized on both sides of a membrane.

osmotic pressure: The pressure exerted by a fluid because of its concentration in solid substances.

Pecquet cistern: A dilated sac at the lower end of the thoracic duct that collects lymph from the lymph capillaries in the lower abdomen. It is also called the large cistern or chyle cistern.

peristalsis: The alternation of contractions and releases of the walls of a hollow organ (vessels, intestines) for the purpose of pushing its contents forward.

Peyer's patches: Groupings of lymphoidal tissue in the mucous membrane that lines the small intestine.

phlebitis: A painful inflammation on the wall of a vein.

physiology: The study of organ function and activity, as opposed to anatomy, which is the study of organ structure.

plasma: The fluid part of blood minus the red blood cells and platelets.

pyruvic acid: Acid created by the breakdown of glucose.

sebaceous gland: A skin gland that expels a fatty substance called sebum.

stasis: The accumulation of fluid when circulation has been slowed or halted.

subclavian: The area beneath the clavicles (or collarbones); the two bones located at the base of the throat.

submandibulary: The area beneath the jawbone.

sudoriferous glands: Skin glands that expel sweat.

terrain: The fluid environment that hosts the cells. The health of the entire body is affected by its good or poor composition.

tonsils: Lymphatic tissue located in the back of the mouth.

toxic substances: Poisonous substances distinguished from toxins by their origin outside the body.

toxins: Wastes and residues created by the body's own metabolism.

triglycerides: Chains of fatty acids.

urea: A toxin created by the breakdown of amino acids that is the chief solid component of urine.

uric acid: Nitrogenous waste present in the urine that is created by the breakdown of proteins.

vacuole: A small cavity or empty space in the tissues containing air or fluid.

valve: A kind of door or portal that opens in only one direction and helps prevent reflux movement of fluid in a vessel.

varicose veins: Abnormal dilation and deformation of a vein.

vasoconstriction: The reduction of the inner space of a vessel by the contraction of its muscle fibers.

villi: Minute, finger-shaped projections in the intestinal mucous membrane that increase the surface area for more efficient food absorption.

Resources

Medicinal Plants

Mountain Rose Herbs offers organic, sustainably sourced products produced in a near-Zero Waste Facility. Contact: 800.879.3337, www.mountainroseherbs.com

Mountain Sage Herbals offers organic, locally sourced, and ethically wildcrafted herbs. Contact: 406.846.4077, www.mountainsageherbals.com

Books

Modern Treatment for Lymphoedema, by Judith Casley-Smith, The Lymphoedema Association of Australia, 5th edition, 1997.

Trampolines

Fitness trampolines, also called rebounders, are available from a variety of vendors. Some things to keep in mind: It is helpful to have one that folds in case you want to travel with it or move it to another space. There are budget models available for about $70, but they may not have the sturdy springs, padded mat, and rebounding action that will be of most benefit.

Clothing

Compression socks and sleeves are available from Absolute Support, Jobst, Juzo, Sigvaris, and Therafirm. They are designed to relieve inflammation and other common symptoms associated with lymphedema and edema. People suffering from poor circulation, deep vein thrombosis (DVT), and leg fatigue also find them helpful, and they are frequently recommended for airplane travel.

Index